Efforts to Make a Difference:

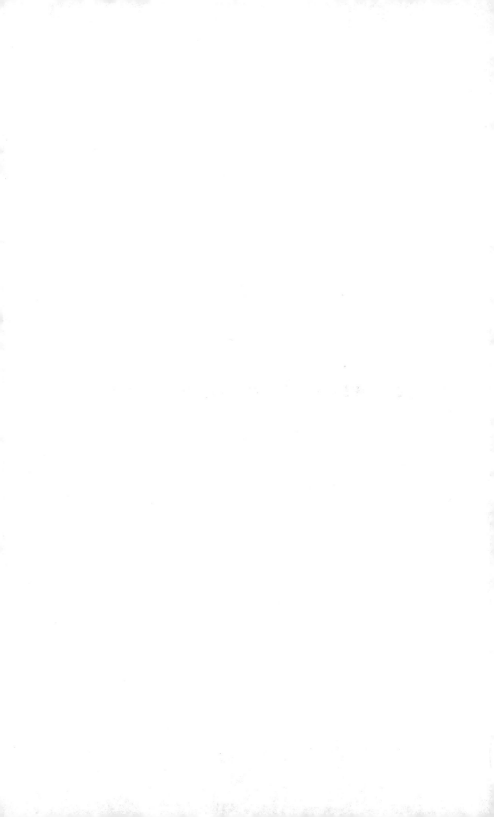

Efforts to Make a Difference:

———⚯———

Reflections of a Hospice Chaplain

Craig L. Falkenstine

Xulon Press

Xulon Press
2301 Lucien Way #415
Maitland, FL 32751
407.339.4217
www.xulonpress.com

Unless otherwise indicated, Scripture quotations taken from the Holy Bible, New Living Translation (NLT). Copyright ©1996, 2004, 2007 by Tyndale House Foundation. Used by permission of Tyndale House Publishers, Inc.

Paperback ISBN-13: 978-1-6628-2452-4
eBook ISBN-13: 978-1-6628-2453-1

This book is dedicated to the memory of
the hospice patients and families I have served,
the hospice workers I have worked beside,
and to my family:

My wife: Ann
My children: Kristy, Mark, Kelly, and Evan
My grandchildren: Zane, Levi, Declan, Asher, Rogan, Myla,
Caden, Felix, and Olivia

Table of Contents

Introduction

———————————⟨◇⟩———————————

There's nothing glamorous about being a hospice chaplain. It's not a job someone dreams about or is excited to become when they grow up. When I was in college, if someone would have said, "You'll be a hospice chaplain someday and work with people who are dying". I would have said, "No way I'd ever do that job!" But the Lord had another plan for me, and this book is a part of that recorded journey and story. It's the Lord preparing my heart and life to serve Him in a unique way of His choosing and the thoughts I learned along the way.

My career as a hospice chaplain was a daily effort to help make a difference in the lives of others as the Lord led me. According to his "big picture" plan, God used my entire life of experiences and relationships, even before He did a work in my heart, to prepare me for what He would work through me in the future. He'll continue to do so until I take my last breath. As I felt led to put this book together, it was for your benefit as the reader, so the Lord could use it in some way to accomplish what only He can accomplish in your heart and through your life.

In this book, I share a variety of special stories of God's work in my life, the insights He taught me, and a few patient stories testifying to God's work in their lives. I've used a modern translation (New Living Translation) of the Bible passages to help readers easily grasp its important truth. This book is meant to be an encouragement to help you see how God can use you to make a meaningful difference in a plan that He has already set in motion.

As you step out in willingness to help others or even seek God, you come with your own set of circumstances that brings with it all your flaws and imperfections. These personal flaws can feed our self-doubts and convince us that you can't do something. We tell ourselves we aren't equipped or simply don't have what it takes." We think God should use someone else who is more qualified. There are many stories of seemingly unequipped people in the Bible who tried to use this excuse with God. But the Lord can equip and uniquely use you because He uniquely created you to bring hope and encouragement to others. But you first must be a willing participant and intentionally submit yourself to be used by God.

The key is learning the first lesson that you aren't expected to be perfect, and the power doesn't come from you alone. You may not be able to see the big picture of your life, but God can. This becomes a matter of faith as you develop a trust in Him to handle the big picture. But you must be willing to be used by God as He chooses in His time. This is what faith in God is all about.

Hebrews 11:6 (NLT)

And it is impossible to please God without faith. Anyone who wants to come to him must believe that God exists and that he rewards those who sincerely seek him.

For me, this collection of testimonies, memories, insights, and short stories is an exercise in preserving some of the many experiences that I didn't want to forget, sharing them as a written testimony of God's handiwork. They are an ongoing written witness to glorify God's awesome work through the power of the Holy Spirit in my life and in my efforts to help others. While sharing some of these special patient stories in this book, I have tried to protect the identities of the patients and families, changing the names of those involved. In the cases where I have identified patients, I have been permitted to do so. Some of these patient stories I wrote years ago, so I wouldn't forget the details of God's providence.

This is not meant to be a best-seller or a major literary work. It's just the opposite: a written record to be passed on to my grandchildren and anyone else who wants to take the time to read my observations and insights.

I pray the Lord will continue to use this book to make a difference through the power of His Holy Spirit in your life. It's a demonstration of what God has done through a changed heart and a willing Christ follower and what He might do in your life and through you if you walk a similar path. I've also included some thoughts and considerations for anyone who might be considering becoming a hospice chaplain.

Some of these experiences are humorous and some sad, but they all demonstrate how the Holy Spirit can work through an individual's life to accomplish something that only God can do. As a hospice chaplain, I was just the vessel that the Lord used at the time, demonstrating that each person is important to God whether they realize it or not.

CHAPTER 1

———⟨✕⟩———

The Beginning of God's Plan to Become a Hospice Chaplain— *Memories of my Grandma, Sarah McGee*

Part of God's preparation for me to become a chaplain and help hospice patients can be traced back to the journey I walked with my grandma, Sarah McGee. Allow me to share with you memories of her that I wanted to preserve. She was the only grandmother I ever knew, and she outlived my mom and dad by many years.

I never knew either of my natural grandmothers because my parents' mothers died long before I was ever born. My mother's father was John Clyde McGee. My grandma called him "Mac." They both lost their first spouses after long illnesses. They met at the old G. C. Murphy's lunch counter on the lower floor on High Street in Morgantown in around 1950. The department store was open early in the mornings to serve breakfast. It had a long bar-like counter with stools located on the lower floor of the department store that was popular back in the day. It had a short-order cook and a waitress, in uniform, who took orders to those seated at the bar.

G. C. Murphy's had a toy department located on that same floor. As a little boy, I loved to go and look at the toys, especially toy cars. I remember being with grandma on one occasion in that toy section when she allowed me to pick out a toy car that she bought for me (Mom had told me not to ask Grandma to buy me anything, but Grandma offered).

My grandfather and grandma met there while they came in every day for breakfast before going to work. My grandfather must have charmed her because he was fifteen years older than her. They fell in love and got married. My mother often said that my grandfather's happiest years were spent with Sarah. Even though she was technically my mother's stepmother, it didn't make any difference with her, and she always claimed my brother and me as her grandchildren, and she was certainly our Grandma McGee.

When I was young, Grandma McGee taught second grade at the old Easton grade school near the intersection of Cheat Road and the Pt. Marion Road. (It was eventually demolished to make way for the new highway.) The last school she taught at before retiring, where she was also the principal, was Morgan Heights Elementary School in Westover, which later became Westwood Medical Clinic on Fairmont Road.

My grandparents lived in the old family house in Woodburn in the city of Morgantown. It had been built in 1923 by my great-grandmother, Mary Catherine (Kate) Brand. The house and property were given to my mom, who was an only child, by her maternal grandmother (Granny) for taking care of her until her death in 1957 at the age of ninety-nine. I still own that house today as a rental property, and it has never left the family. My parents (Gerald and Clarice Falkenstine) built a new home on the lower side of the property in 1950, and my grandparents lived in the old house behind us when I was young. I have an older brother, Brett, and I came along in 1954.

I was in and out of my grandparents' house about every day, and my mother often thought I was being a pest to them. They often sat in yard chairs in the summertime and watched us play. My grandmother kept all kinds of jellies (many of them home-made) on the kitchen table with bread, so they were always ready for a snack. I know my grandfather enjoyed it. I would bring her grapes from my other grandfather's house, from which she made wonderful jelly.

My grandparents had a dark-blue Pontiac convertible that I enjoyed riding around in with the top down. Maybe that's why I have a convertible today. To a little kid who has always loved cars, riding with the top down was the coolest thing ever. Grandma told me that I knew every kind of car on the road by the time I was four years old. That old Pontiac had an Indian hood ornament that lit up when the lights were turned on. I remember getting in trouble for turning the headlights on in the garage and running the battery down because I wanted to see that hood ornament light up.

Grandma took me with her to her class at Easton school on two occasions when I was five years old and before I started school. She took me with her on Halloween, so I could wear my costume and see the bigger kids parade around in their costumes. I also was there for May Day (no one knows what that is today) and saw the girls dance around the maypole. It was interesting seeing my grandmother as the take-charge teacher in the classroom.

Grandma often talked about all the teeth that she had pulled out for the young kids in her classroom when it was time for them to lose their front teeth. When it was time for me to lose my front teeth, I wouldn't let my parents touch them. I wanted someone who was experienced and that meant Grandma.

On Halloween night in 1961, when I was seven years old, I went trick or treating in our neighborhood. My last stop before going home was my grandparents' house. That night my grandfather anxiously waited for me to come, so he could see me. Grandma greeted me at the door while my grandfather greeted me from the top of the steps. He wasn't feeling well and went to bed as soon as I left. He died of an apparent heart attack that night right in front of my grandmother. My grandmother screamed for my mother to come, but he was already gone. They told me the next morning that Grandpa McGee had died. That was my first experience with death.

My parents made a poor choice and tried to protect me rather than letting me experience the funeral home visitation and funeral. I had no clue about any of that. I remember going up to my grandparents' house the next day to see grandma. She was sitting in a chair and immediately patted the tops of her thighs with both hands, then opened her arms for me to come sit on her lap, so she could talk to me. It was so comforting to me.

Grandma decided she wanted to buy her own little house in Westover near her new school, where she was now the principal as well as a teacher. I would visit her regularly at her new house with Mom. We loved sitting on the swing on her back porch, which overlooked her backyard. She loved watching the birds, and she fed them every day after she retired in 1972.

After my grandfather died, my grandmother traded in her old Pontiac convertible and got a light-blue 1961 Ford Falcon. In 1967 my dad bought a Ford Mustang, and in 1968 Grandma decided she wanted to buy a new car. She talked with my dad, wanting to know what kind of car would hold its value, seeing as her Falcon had not. Dad told her that the new "pony cars"—Mustangs, Camaros, and other sporty cars—would hold their value since they were so popular. So, to our surprise, Grandma ordered herself a new Chevrolet Camaro. It was red with a white racing stripe and a red interior with bucket seats. She ordered a six-cylinder engine with an automatic transmission, no power steering or brakes, and stock hubcaps. That was her last car, which she kept for almost thirty years. I had the rust repaired and painted for her back in the 1980s. When she decided to stop driving in her eighties, she wanted that Camaro to sit in her carport, so she could just look at it. She loved it when young men commented on it and offered to buy it. She often told me she was surprised when people offered her more money for it than she had paid for it. My dad was right; it was a good value.

My dad died suddenly of a heart attack in 1969 when I was fifteen years old. My mom had struggled and grieved when my grandfather died eight years earlier. Now in her late forties and suddenly finding herself a widow, she went to pieces. My grandmother took on a new role with my mother and was a stabilizing force in her life. She talked with her often. Grandma was a stabilizer in all our lives. She had a very even-tempered personality and showed little emotion other than laughter, but she was very empathetic. Maybe that's why she was a good schoolteacher and Sunday school teacher and weathered so many storms in her own life.

Grandma was a strong Christian. Her mother had died when she was a girl, and she was raised by her grandmother. Her father died, and then her grandmother, and she lived with an aunt, if I remember correctly. She got married young and had three children. Her first husband had kidney disease and died in 1948. Two of her three children inherited the same kidney disease and died as young adults. She had been through many storms in her life, so her faith was especially important to her.

After college I moved away and started a job in Indiana, PA, and then moved to Johnstown, PA, in time to be there for the 1977 Johnstown Flood that killed ninety people. I had never seen such devastation. While I was in Johnstown, I accepted Jesus Christ as my savior, and the Lord began working in my heart. When I told my grandmother that I had accepted Christ, she said she had always been praying for the salvation of her grandchildren (my testimony is in the following chapter).

I moved back to Morgantown in 1980 when my mother started having health issues. I was also in the process of trying to get a new radio station on the air in Morgantown. While in the hospital, Mom accepted Jesus Christ and found peace before dying suddenly in 1982. I was living in an apartment in my Grandfather Falkenstine's old house, which my uncle had made into apartments. I had gone over to my mom's house to pick up my mail. She was living in the old family house that Grandma and Grandpa McGee had lived in but which had been remodeled. I was in a hurry that day to go (I wanted to call some girl for a date), but my mother said she wanted to talk with me. "You never take time to talk with me anymore," she said. I told mom that tomorrow I would come by her house after work, and we'd talk then. Mom had the saddest look on her face as she stood at the front door when I left.

The next day I came by, but Mom wasn't home. It made me mad that she wasn't there because I had told her I was coming by after work. When I got to my apartment, my answering machine was full of messages from the hospital emergency room trying to find me. My mom had gone out shopping and suddenly dropped dead of a heart attack on the sidewalk while walking back to her car. I knew the man who saw her fall, and he told me she was dead before she hit the sidewalk. He and the EMS squad did CPR, but she never revived.

It took me a while to deal with myself. I had to ask the Lord to forgive me, but the biggest issue was learning to forgive myself. Why didn't I take the time to talk with my mother that day when she wanted to talk with me? What did she want to talk to me about? I retold that story of coming to the place where I could forgive myself many times to people over the years as I counseled them. The Lord helped me heal and work through that issue. He has used my retelling of that story to help other folks deal with the struggle to forgive themselves when their loved ones have died or were dying.

I went to my grandmother's house to tell her that Mom had died. I anticipated that I would be the one comforting her because she would have to go through yet another death, but she was the one who comforted me. When I sat down on the couch next to her and told her what happened, she put her arms around me, and I just lost it. I was once again being comforted by my grandmother just as she had done when my grandfather died. She continued to be very comforting to my brother and me as we went through that time.

I remember going to visit my grandmother after mom died. I was in my twenties, but I felt like an adult orphan. My grandmother continued to serve as our family "anchor," providing a family connection that was important to me. She reassured me and provided emotional support, probably without realizing it. Whenever I went to visit her, as I was leaving, she would come to the front picture window and wave goodbye until I was out of sight. I remember thinking, *"What will I do when she dies?"*

As a young man in college (West Virginia University), I was the first university student to be elected to Morgantown City Council. I ran for mayor in 1976 and lost by one vote on city council. I also ran for county magistrate in 1976 and made a decent showing but lost that election too. After that election my grandmother said to me, "Promise me you won't run for any more political offices again." I asked why, and she told me that she didn't want me going in as an honest person and coming out corrupted. As I observe the world and politics now, I can see why she said that.

Grandma approved of my wife, Ann, who was a nurse when we got married. It was special when Grandma asked if I would like to have my grandfather's wedding band as my wedding band. I was thrilled to have that wedding ring, and that gesture is one of the most cherished things I remember my grandmother doing for me. I still wear that wedding band and have asked the Lord to help me find it more than twice when I have lost it.

After I got married, sometimes Grandma would call our house and ask to talk with Ann rather than me. Grandma often ran all her medical issues past Ann to get her opinion. Ann would also take Grandma to appointments. Grandma enjoyed our kids, and I was thankful I had someone to call to report about their birth. I would always go and pick up Grandma to come to our house for Christmas Eve dinner, and she would give the kids their first Christmas presents. Then we all then went to church for the Christmas Eve candlelight service.

When her health began to decline, she announced that only her great-grandchildren would receive gifts because it was too much to keep track of. Grandma was also well known for her homemade Christmas tree ornaments, which she gave away. When my daughter Kelly's boyfriend, Cameron, (now her husband) came to our house at Christmas time, he mentioned he had an ornament on his tree that he got as a little boy, just like the one we had on our tree. It turns out he had been in my grandmother's Sunday school class at Crescent Hills Bible Chapel as a little boy and had gotten one.

Grandma was diagnosed with colon cancer. She had a major colon surgery requiring a colostomy and needed to learn how to deal with the bag appliances that would hold her waste. The doctors were amazed at how quickly she learned and adjusted. She told me that when she was young, she wanted to go to college and become a doctor, but she was told women don't become doctors. People said if she wanted to go to college, she could go and become a teacher. So, that's what she did, earning a master's degree in education as well.

Grandma decided not to have any chemo and lived three quality years independently in her own home (with her only living child, Ed Robey, and his wife, Thelma, living next door) before the cancer returned. She didn't want to have any surgery or chemo, but the surgeon, whom she liked, convinced her that it was necessary because the cancer was approaching her spine, and the pain would be difficult to manage. She had a twelve-hour surgery, and everyone was surprised a ninety-year-old could survive it all. While recuperating at Ruby Memorial Hospital, she had a heart attack and spent the next few weeks declining, with dementia now taking over.

Ann and I were at the hospital every day keeping track of her condition and advising Ed about what needed to be done. My brother flew up from Houston to see her, knowing this would be the last time he would see her alive. She recognized him but was extremely uncomfortable, so he spent the night with her in the hospital to help meet her needs. I had grown accustomed to knowing what she needed and knew how to adjust her bed when she made certain motions with her hand. During the night when Brett couldn't figure out what she was trying to tell him, she finally said, "Where's Craig? He knows what I need." I think Brett was more emotional about saying goodbye to Grandma than he was when our parents died.

My main prayer request every day to the Lord that summer was that I wanted to be with Grandma when she died. Because of my parents' sudden deaths, I had a need in my heart to be with her when she died. Little did I know how this experience would change the course of my life. The Lord used it to send me on a different path to become a chaplain.

I was at the hospital every day after work and on weekends. Because of her dementia and severe hearing loss, she became difficult with the staff, but she always knew me. She imagined at times she was back in the classroom playing teacher or principal. If she thought the staff weren't asking respectfully or using proper grammar, she would order them to leave the room. I would go in some days, and the nurse would tell me that Grandma had thrown out the doctor, the physical therapist, or nurse who didn't ask nicely or properly that day. I remember an intern coming into the room while I was there who was almost shaking when he said, "I need to draw her blood. What should I do?" I told him to ask for permission. He would need to talk into a microphone that was connected to a headset over her ears, so she could hear. So, he said, "May I please draw your blood?"

"What for?" Grandma asked. He gave her a medical explanation that she appreciated, and all was well. I remember her saying to me one time, "Craig, they have given me five CAT scans. Why on earth does anyone need five CAT scans?" All I could say was that I didn't know.

On a Thursday in August 1998, the doctors told us that she had only twenty-four hours to live. We had already paid to go away for the weekend to Canaan Valley for a family Sunday school retreat. I decided I would stay behind and maybe come up later if/when Grandma passed.

Friday turned into Saturday, which turned into Sunday, which turned into Monday, and the doctors were still saying she had twenty-four hours to live. When Tuesday came, I went into the hospital early to check on her before I went to my office In Uniontown, PA. I told the nurse what my prayer request was, to be with Grandma when she died. "She has fooled us all weekend," the nurse said, "but I'll call you with any changes."

At about 9:30 a.m., the nurse called me at the office and told me there were some changes in Grandma's vital signs and that she would keep me posted. I needed to take care of some things in the office in case I couldn't come back the next day and spent another forty-five minutes taking care of the details. Then I told our receptionist that I was going back to the hospital in Morgantown.

It was a beautiful summer day, and during the forty-minute drive from Uniontown to Morgantown, I felt peaceful and calm. This was before the days of cell phones, so I didn't know that as soon as I left the office, the nurse had called saying I needed to come to the hospital immediately if I wanted to see my grandmother alive.

Not realizing what was going on, I took my time and parked my new car, so no one would bang my doors in the hospital parking lot. I used the bathroom and got a drink of water, wasting all this time not knowing what was going on. As soon as the nurse saw me, she said, "Your grandmother is dying."

I walked up to Grandma's bedside, took her hand, and said, "I'm here, Grandma." Immediately, she took her last breath.

The Lord immediately spoke to my heart and said, "I got you here for the minute." The moment had the Lord's signature all over it. He had answered my prayer, and I knew it. Grandma was now with my grandfather and my parents in heaven.

The Lord used Grandma to teach me one last lesson. He started me on a new course in life with her death where I became a hospice chaplain and pastoral counselor. Grandma, as a teacher, would have been pleased that she had taught me that final lesson. I used all my bereavement experiences with my parents and grandparents to help others deal with death and dying. I also became one of the founders of the West Virginia Family Grief Center, where I'm still the president of the board. The non-profit grief center works with children and families who have lost loved ones.

I thank God for the lady who wasn't my natural grandmother but who was even more special because of her commitment to our family long after my grandfather died. She was the only grandmother I ever knew, my Grandma McGee.

CHAPTER 2

———◇———

My Personal Testimony: Jesus Making a Difference

It's interesting to look back at what the Lord has done in my life, to put my personal history into writing to see how the Lord put together all the pieces of the puzzle of my life. This story intersects with the story of my grandmother and the Lord's call on my life.

Growing up, my family consisted of my mom and dad (Gerald and Clarice Falkenstine) and my older brother, Brett. We lived in Morgantown, the home of West Virginia University, a town with a population of approximately 35,000 in northern West Virginia. I went to church my entire life, always wearing a tie, sport coat, and shoes that were reserved for Sundays and other special occasions. That was the dress norm of the day. My dad was the chairman of the board of the Methodist Church we attended, taught an adult Sunday school class, and believed we all were to be in church each week—no matter what. My mom taught the kindergarten class during Sunday school time and tended not to have much interest in spiritual matters or Christians she viewed as fanatical hypocrites. Brett

13

just moaned and groaned that he had to go, especially as he became a teenager.

Life seemed pretty normal except during those times when my mother was sick and would be in the hospital for long periods of time. In those days, kids weren't allowed in for visitation, so there were times when I could only see my mom through the hospital room window, waving to me several stories below. I remember being prepared in the fourth grade that she might not come home. But she did come home, although she never seemed to be in good health and was very fragile, emotional, and often cranky.

My dad was the rock of our family in his quiet but firm manner. Although I didn't share his love of baseball, he still spent time with me and regularly did things that I wanted to do. We usually had some sort of Sunday afternoon ritual that always ended by going over to visit my grandfather (my dad's father). Grandpa Hank always had a new box of animal crackers for me to eat while he and dad visited, and grandpa smoked his pipe.

I have always loved cars. Each fall my Dad would take me around every new car lot in town, so I could look at all the new models and collect new car brochures. I still have many of them today. Some of them are over fifty years old and have some value. He would endure the endless sales pitches, so I could look at the new cars and keep my collection up to date.

When I was older, I had a go-cart that the two of us would take out on Sundays to a shopping plaza to run (back then stores were closed on Sundays). The big thrill came the summer I was fifteen years old, and he taught me, in that same shopping plaza parking lot, how to drive his sporty 1967 Mustang with its manual transmission. I was so excited because, in a few months, I would be sixteen and could get my driver's license.

My dad was never sick and seemed to handle life without too much difficulty, even when it was difficult. Then, in the fall of my sophomore year in high school in 1969, my dad died suddenly of a heart attack. That was the day my childhood came to a screeching halt, and I was forced to grow up quickly.

My mother did not cope well after my father's death. She had never worked and had quit college to marry Dad. She never even balanced the checkbook. My dad did everything. To top things off, Brett was leaving for Vietnam within a few months. Mom started drinking more and more until she became an alcoholic over the course of two years. It wasn't until a bleeding ulcer put her back in the hospital that she was forced to "dry out."

Grandpa Hank (William Harvey Falkenstine) outlived my dad and became an important, emotional connection for me to my dad, as did my relationships with my uncles. I visited Grandpa weekly, took his laundry to him, did all his shopping, and willingly chauffeured him anywhere he wanted to go. He even had me cut his hair and do many of the things my dad had done for him. I was nineteen when Grandpa Hank died, also of a sudden heart attack. Once again my world was rocked by grief and loss.

Brett made it back from Vietnam safely and then moved away to Illinois to get his master's degree. While there he met a girl named Linda who called herself a Christian. Brett made fun of her religion even though they liked each other. Through their relationship journey, the Lord was finally able to draw Brett to Himself while he was in Washington, DC.

One afternoon Brett said he wanted to have lunch together, so we could talk. We met at a fast-food restaurant in between my college classes at West Virginia University. That's when he dropped the bombshell. I thought he had fallen off the deep end. He had become what he used to make fun of—a born-again Christian. I just wrote it off for love. He and Linda were finally going to get married. They had dedicated their lives to Christ and determined they would have a celibate lifestyle until they got married. I found all this rather humorous although our mother did not. She thought Linda was not a suitable mate for her eldest son. Brett's new faith challenged me. Although interested, I decided that giving up partying and living a moral lifestyle was not for me.

Following their wedding, Brett and Linda moved to Houston, Texas. I graduated from college and eventually moved about two hours north of my hometown. It was close enough that I could still keep tabs on Mom but far enough that I could have a life of my own. Little did I know what the Lord had in store for me.

The job I had accepted was to replace a guy who was a born-again Christian who felt called into the ministry. I spent a lot of time with this guy for two weeks to learn his position. It was the first time I was able to closely observe someone who lived as a Christian and had an actual relationship with Jesus. I found it rather scary and challenging, but my love for sin was still much greater than my desire to give my life to Jesus.

Almost two more years went by. I moved to Johnstown, PA, just in time to experience the 1977 Johnstown Flood, which killed over ninety people. I had never experienced such disaster, devastation, and death. A spiritual awakening began to happen in Johnstown as that town tried to rebuild and deal with this major "act of God."

By then I had branched off and started my own advertising agency, bought my first old house (for $20,000), which was an old duplex with a rental property, and had a new car every year. I was also beginning to realize that all the things I thought would fill the void in my heart did not. I wasn't married yet and was following all the ways of the world in the wrong direction.

My life goal in 1978 was to build my own radio station back in my hometown of Morgantown. I met several people who had the engineering capability and connections to help me secure a new radio frequency for the Morgantown area and to put a new radio station on the air. This process involved petitioning the FCC for rulemaking procedures, which ended up being a long, drawn-out, and expensive procedure that took a few years.

One day I went to see a friend who was a radio station DJ. He was intelligent, quick-witted, and could tell the best dirty jokes. Because of the advertising agency, he would often record radio commercials for me. But something had happened to him. He was drastically different.

"What's new?" I asked.

"Craig, Jesus is what's new," he replied. He told me that he came home one day and found a note from his Christian wife saying she couldn't take it anymore and had moved out. He was crushed. He planned to commit suicide, but he cried out to God, saying if God was real, he wanted Jesus to come into his life. He said it was as if someone had dumped a bucket of warm water over him. The Lord changed his heart, and I could see the positive, radical change in his life, right before my eyes. I was fascinated by his conversion and how he was processing his new faith. He gave me all these interesting cartoon tracts to read and started dragging me to a charismatic prayer meeting on Tuesday nights. They sure weren't like the Methodists I had known growing up!

On the second Tuesday night meeting I attended, the Lord convicted my heart to the point that I caved in and gave my heart to Christ. I was born again on February 27, 1979. The pastor had asked anyone who would like to accept Jesus as their Savior to raise their hand. Nervously and cautiously, I raised my hand. That night after the meeting, I was telling a new Christian friend that I thought some sort of bell or whistle would go off in my mind, but I didn't feel any different, so I doubted my salvation. My new friend opened the Bible to Romans 10:9 – 10, which says, "That if you confess with your mouth, 'Jesus is Lord,' and believe in your heart that God raised him from the dead, you will be saved. For it is with your heart that you believe and are justified, and it is with your mouth that you confess and are saved."

In reading that scripture, the Lord allowed me to clearly see my salvation. The Lord used this scripture as a rock for me to step out in faith. This was the first step toward building a new foundation in the Lord for my life. I never doubted my salvation again.

2 Corinthians 5:17 (NLT)

This means that anyone who belongs to Christ has become a new person. The old life is gone; a new life has begun.

In spring 1979, the TV series *Jesus of Nazareth* was showing on TV. My old friends came by my house, with six-packs of beer to party with me. They were dumbfounded that I wanted to watch *Jesus of Nazareth* rather than party with them. The Lord provided a whole new set of Christian friends that mentored and discipled me in many ways during the following months.

When I telephoned Brett to tell him the news, he was thrilled and told me that he had been praying daily for me. The next person I had to tell was my mother. Oh, how I dreaded that. What would she say with two religious fanatics for sons?

My mother listened to my story and conversion, but more importantly, she watched my life and saw that I no longer was doing the things I used to do. I began to pray earnestly for her salvation. I also began to wonder about my dad's spiritual state. It was frightening to think that maybe my dad had gone through all the motions of thinking he was Christian but had never formally accepted Christ. Growing up in our church, I couldn't remember hearing any type of salvation message. My dad didn't smoke or drink, and he didn't even swear when he got mad. I knew from his life and the type of books that he read that he was searching. I wished I knew where he stood with the Lord when he died.

Within a year of my conversion, my mom's doctor called me and said he thought my mom might have cancer. He wanted her to go to the hospital for some tests, but she had refused. He hoped she would listen to me. I had already sold my home in Pennsylvania, so I moved back to Morgantown, expecting the worst when mom went into the hospital. She wanted a private room, but they were all full, so she had to settle for a semi-private room.

Mom's new hospital roommate was a born-again Christian lady from the Morgantown Christian & Missionary Alliance Church. She and my mother hit it off right away. As the woman's pastor (Doug Miller) came to visit her daily for the next two weeks, he developed a relationship with my mom as well. At the end of those two weeks, he had the privilege of praying with and leading mom to Christ. As it turned out, mom got better and didn't have cancer, but I thank God for the circumstances that led her to the Lord.

Mom and I began attending the CMA church, where we met several families we had known from our old church, who were now at CMA. One of those couples, John E. and Bonnie

Pyles, told me a story I'll forever be grateful for (later this couple filled in as my parents in my wedding). John said that about two weeks before my dad died, he and Bonnie had a Bible study in their home, led by a couple who had been conducting lay witness revivals in Methodist churches. My dad had accepted Christ at their Bible Study just two weeks before he died suddenly of a heart attack. Hallelujah! I finally knew Dad's story. Mom later commented that she had seen a change in Dad during a trip they had taken to Baltimore a few days later, shortly before his death.

Now my mom was going to a women's Bible study and even attended a Bible study I taught, always with all her homework done. Two years after Mom accepted Christ, she died suddenly from a heart attack while shopping. How grateful I am for God's grace in allowing Mom and Dad to accept his gift of salvation before they died.

I met my wife at the CMA church within two weeks of mom's death, and we were eventually married there. Two of our children were also married there, and later I became an elder and was head elder for almost ten years. I thank God for His love, grace, and providence in our lives.

My dream of starting the radio station became a reality in 1982, and it's still on the air today as WZST (100.9 FM). I seemed to pray my way through all the struggles and stress, so I originally gave the radio station the call letters WJCF. They stood for Jesus and Craig Falkenstine. I was certain the radio station would be a success because I was Christian, and God would be on my side and give me what I wanted. I thought God was going to do all of this for me.

But it wasn't a financial success. It was a financial failure that took almost all the money I had inherited and borrowed. I had no choice but to get out of the radio station. My dream had gone down the tubes. I didn't understand why the Lord would bring me through all of that, only to lose the radio station of my dreams in the end. It was depressing. I was married, and we were expecting a new baby, and I had no career. Later, I discovered that when you walk with the Lord, failure doesn't define you. It becomes a new means for the Lord to redirect your life according to His will. Adversity is certainly a refining process in our relationship with the Lord. It's during difficult times that we learn the most about trusting the Lord.

Eventually, I went to work for a new home health agency to handle public relations. Little did I know that my new field of endeavor would evolve into a career that would last for the next thirty-five years. When I started in home health, the position of a hospice chaplain didn't even exist. However, the Lord was once again "working all things out for good" according to His will for the future. As time went on, I saw the new hospice program begin and grow out of the home health program. The national Medicare hospice program was started, and our company began to develop a Medicare-certified hospice program as well. This new program began hiring chaplains and all the necessary staff. Someone once said, "When the Lord closes one door, He opens a new one." After seeing a training film, I thought I'd love to be a hospice chaplain.

After my parents' death, my grandmother was an important person in my life. She was the last connection to my childhood other than my brother. Following her illness and death, I began my journey to become a hospice chaplain and start a bereavement ministry. I attained the necessary credentials and degree to become a chaplain while working with the home health and hospice agency. Two years later, I received a certification in pastoral counseling. Upon completion, I was able to step into the role of a chaplain within the same company.

When I was a boy, I had a paper route and had to collect money for the newspapers I delivered. My older customers loved me because I would visit and patiently sit and listen to them talk. My wife says that was the preparation I needed for listening to people as a chaplain and pastoral counselor. The Lord had prepared me with a heart for hurting people who had lost loved ones as well as caring for those who are terminally ill. I spent the remainder of my career as a hospice chaplain and counselor, working with terminally ill individuals and their families. I also helped start the West Virginia Grief Center, a non-profit organization, in 2002. It continues to provide peer support to grieving families with children. It also has a community bereavement support group that anyone can attend. I'm still president of the board of directors.

Romans 8:28 became my life verse, helping me realize that God can use even the most hurtful and sad times of life to prepare us for a meaningful ministry. It's definitely a "God thing" where both the bad and good circumstances of my life can be used in a positive way to help others in God's will. This life preparation gave me the credibility to minister to hurting people. As CMA pastor A.W. Tozer once said, "It is doubtful whether God can bless a man until he has hurt him deeply. I like the modern version: "God doesn't greatly bruise someone before he can greatly use someone."

Romans 8:28 (NLT)

And we know that God causes everything to work together for the good of those who love God and are called according to his purpose for them.

Patient Stories:

CHAPTER 3

———————⚬———————

Maybe I'll See the Chaplain

As a chaplain I needed to respect and honor where people were at in their personal walk with God, no matter what they believed. I could never get on a soapbox and preach at them or tell them they were wrong. Many times, people who called themselves atheists or were of a religion other than Christianity simply declined to see the chaplain, and I never met with them. It was their right to decline chaplain services. But sometimes the Lord arranged divine opportunities. Some of the stories I will share illustrate God's hand in such situations. Regardless of each patients' desires, I always knew who each patient was and their medical condition in case a need developed.

Whenever I met a new patient and his or her family, I knew it was important to develop a trusting, personal relationship with them. Even if I greatly disagreed with them or thought they were wrong, I respected them and their beliefs. Developing a relationship was an important first step to gaining trust with patients and families. Many times, with frequent visits to see patients just for socialization over time, they came to trust me as the visiting chaplain, and I became their friend. They felt comfortable and felt safe enough to ask me meaningful questions about God, the Bible, and going to heaven. I needed them to reach the point where God was drawing their hearts to Himself, and they were personally searching for an accurate, biblical answer. I would always offer to pray aloud for the patients I visited, and most usually accepted my offer. It became a meaningful time in our relationship. Occasionally, some patients declined my offer to pray for them, and I respected their wishes.

We all were created with a place in our heart reserved for a one-on-one relationship with God, but many times we choose to fill that "God-shaped void" with something else. No family members can decide for us to follow Jesus, nor can anyone force us to believe. God loves us and gives us a free will to choose whether to love Him in return. Again, God doesn't want us to have religion but a personal, daily relationship with Him, a meaningful connection to Him in our lives that only comes by having that one-on-one, growing relationship with Jesus Christ .

I used to tell patients that going to church or church membership alone doesn't make you a Christian any more than walking into a garage makes you a Cadillac. God knows our hearts.

We admitted an elderly man with liver failure into hospice. When the nurse asked if he wanted to see the chaplain, his answer was "Maybe." When I would call him, he would always tell me, "Maybe I could come some other time," but he never said no.

After a few weeks, the nurse came to me and said the patient was very jaundiced, declining quickly, and she sensed he needed to talk with me. I called him and said, "I'd like to come to see you at 1:00 today. Is that, OK?" He said I could come. He lived out in the country in a simple small home with his wife, who was his caregiver.

It was summertime, and we visited on his small back porch. I sat across from him with our knees close to each other because of the space restrictions. He was very jaundiced looking in his eyes and skin, having the typical yellow coloring that told the story of his diagnosis. With any first chaplain visit, it was always important for me to get to know the patient and his or her family and allow the patient to tell me his or her personal story. It always painted a picture of who they were, what they believed, and why they believed it.

This patient sat across from me with his arms folded across his chest in a very defensive posture, which told me a lot. He proceeded to tell me that his brother-in-law was a preacher and had told him for the last forty years that he was going to hell because he didn't go to church. I told him my saying: "Going to church doesn't make you a Christian any more than walking into a garage makes you a Cadillac." Although, I think I substituted "pickup truck" for "Cadillac" because I thought he could identify more with that. That seemed to hit home with him.

"Yeah, that's right," he said.

I was now his friend, and his countenance changed as he unfolded his arms. He proceeded to tell me that he had actually accepted Christ as his Savior at a vacation Bible school when he was a boy. He seemed to avoid church out of rebellion because of his brother-in-law's position and holier-than-thou attitude.

We talked for a while until it was obvious that he wasn't feeling well and wanted to go to bed. I asked if I could pray for him, and he agreed. I leaned forward and rested my arms on my thighs with my hands and fingers intertwined and prayed for him as the Lord led me. Suddenly, he leaned forward and grabbed my hands as if he were hanging on for dear life and became very emotional. As best as I could determine, he got his heart right with the Lord that afternoon. When I left, I told him I would be back to see him on Monday.

When I arrived on Monday, he was in a coma and had not been out of bed since I saw him on Friday. He died later that day. Afterwards, I had the chance to talk with his adult children and his wife. They asked if I would do a graveside service for him, which I did. I also had the opportunity to visit later with his family and saw his wife in the nursing home in later years. I had the opportunity to pray and visit with her until her death. God had his fingerprints of love all over this patient.

CHAPTER 4

———————⋈———————

I'm Not Dead Yet!

On Valentine's Day, 2005, I did the funeral for an eighty-six-year-old man, whom I'll call Arthur, at a funeral home in Preston County. Exactly eight months earlier to the day, on June 14, 2004, I was told that Arthur needed to see me immediately. I went to his house, which was a three-room shack with running water only in the kitchen sink and no bathroom. They used a port-a-john next to the house as an outhouse. My previous visits to his house were on his old front porch, but that day Arthur was in bed and wasn't feeling well.

Arthur's ex-wife, who I'll call Sissy, was there along with her mother. Arthur told me he had married Sissy many years earlier when she got pregnant by another man to make her an "honest woman." He was about forty-three years older than her. Things hadn't gone well, and they divorced many years ago. Now she was back taking care of him, and he wanted her to have whatever of his Supplemental Security Income (SSI) or insurance she could have after he died. To facilitate this, he wanted to marry her again, and he wanted me to do the wedding. When I asked him when he wanted me to do it, he said, "Now," because he didn't have much time left.

I informed him that to get married, he needed a marriage license. So, at Arthur's insistence, I took Sissy in my Jeep to the courthouse. Poor Sissy stunk to high heaven in the June heat as we made our way to the courthouse. She had little education and couldn't read or write. Her conversations amounted to being brief answers to whatever questions I asked.

She had cash in hand, and she paid the fees to get the marriage application. However, she couldn't get the license until she had Arthur's signature on it as well. So, we made the fifteen-mile drive back to Arthur's shack.

It soon became clear that Sissy couldn't even begin filling out the marriage license. So, our social worker, who was sitting with Arthur until we got back, helped Sissy with it. After getting Arthur's signature, we drove fifteen miles back to the courthouse. Sissy obtained the license, and we were on the road again.

We finally made it back to the shack for me to do my first-ever marriage for a hospice patient who was remarrying his ex-wife, an ex-wife who was forty-three years younger than him. Arthur was fast asleep when we arrived. He was in his bed with dirty sheets that looked like they had never been washed. Finally, we were able to wake him long enough to sit on the edge of the bed to get married. The witnesses were a neighbor girl and Sissy's mother, who just shook her head the whole time I was there.

The next time I saw Arthur, he was living in an old, rented trailer that our social services staff had encouraged the couple to move into. At least the trailer had a bathroom with running water so our aides could give him a bath. The windows in the trailer were wide open with no easy way to close them. Sissy and her mother sat in front of a TV, which was in front of the A/C, which ran even though the windows were stuck open. That day Arthur was able to sit at the kitchen table and talk— or, rather, complain.

A few days after that visit, I was headed to Bridgeport for an IDG (inter-disciplinary group) meeting when I got a call from our home health aide. "Arthur says he's dying and wants to see you as quickly as possible," he said.

When I arrived, Sissy and her mother were calmly watching TV and said Arthur was in the bedroom. The aide had stayed with Arthur until I arrived. He told me that Arthur had said, "The Lord's going to take me today."

In the tiny bedroom, Arthur took my hand and held it as he asked me if I would "preach" his funeral and make sure Sissy was taken care of. Then he asked me to pray for him. When I was finished, Arthur closed his eyes, took a deep breath, and let it out as if he were going to die immediately. He laid there a few moments, keeping his eyes tightly closed while holding his breath and my hand. Then he peeked out of one eye and said, "I'm not dead yet." He seemed surprised that he hadn't died, as he had expected.

The nurse came and examined him, then mouthed the words "He's fine" to me. All his vital signs were normal, and his blood pressure was better than mine that day. She asked him when was the last time he had eaten anything. "This morning," he replied. He said he had eaten two eggs, toast, bacon, and coffee. He had eaten a bigger breakfast than I did. It was all too obvious that Arthur only thought he was dying that day. He said repeatedly that he thought for sure that the Lord was taking him home that day. I left and told him I would see him again later. I went back to the office and told everyone what had happened.

Later that night Arthur telephoned the owner of the funeral home telling him to come and get him because he was dying. He had made arrangements with the funeral director for his funeral several years before. "I've never had a hospice patient call me themselves to come and get them," the funeral director said. He was a little confused and amused at the thought. The funeral director called our hospice office and heard my story from the nursing supervisor and laughed. He said he'd go and visit Arthur, but he wouldn't take his cart.

A few weeks later, Arthur got worse and had to go live in a nursing home. The last couple of times I saw Arthur, he didn't know me and was out of it. When Arthur died I talked with the funeral director regarding the details of my doing Arthur's funeral, as he had requested.

Arthur, as a corpse, was well dressed in a suit and tie and, uncharacteristically, looked sharp and dignified. I told the funeral director that he looked great but that he never looked that good in life. The funeral director said Arthur came with no clothes, so the funeral director had given him one of his old suits, shirt, and tie, so he would look nice. Arthur had planned his funeral and assigned a life-insurance policy over to the funeral home to make sure the costs were covered. The funeral director said it didn't cover the entire cost, but it was close enough.

Arthur's service was in the funeral home's large main room, which could easily have held one hundred people, even though only five were in attendance. Other than Sissy and her mother, two of Arthur's nephews came to the service. The fifth person at the service was someone who didn't even know Arthur, but Sissy had gotten him to drive Arthur's old five-speed car to get her and her mother to the service.

Sissy cried the entire time. Her mother, who seemed to have some form of dementia, talked loudly before and throughout the service, even during my first prayer. It seemed as if she were doing color commentary for Sissy, as if the funeral were a sporting event. "Here comes the preacher," she'd say. "He's going to pray now." Then, "He's done praying now." This type of commentary went on throughout the service and was very distracting at the time but very humorous as I look back on it now.

At least Sissy and her mother had both taken a bath before coming. Sissy was wearing old dirty tennis shoes, brown socks, grey pants, a T-shirt, and a navy blue zip-up sweatshirt. Her mother was wearing blue pants, a blue top, and a plaid hunting shirt.

As the two-car funeral procession reached the cemetery, the funeral director and I, along with the gravediggers, got the coffin over to the grave for me to do the typical graveside committal service.

No one got out of the other car, so the funeral director walked over to see if anyone wanted to be there for the committal service. Reluctantly, Sissy got out and came over as I did the short service. As soon as I said, "Amen," Sissy ran to the car, jumped in, and the car sped off as if they had just robbed the bank. I turned to the funeral director. "What was that all about?" I asked. "Did they think you were going to hand them a bill?" The story of Arthur and his family was one of those patient stories that I'll never forget.

CHAPTER 5

———————∞———————

My Uncle's Long-Lost Friend

In the early days of hospice in our area, I was the only chaplain for a company in West Virginia that had hospice offices in Morgantown, Bridgeport, and Wheeling. Because there were a small total number of hospice patients, I would work out of the three offices in three different cities. I would start my day at the Morgantown office on certain days, then I'd start in Bridgeport on other days, making the forty-mile trip back and forth in addition to driving all over the different counties, going wherever patients lived. I could easily do over one hundred miles a day. Every other week I would get up at the crack of dawn and drive one and a half hours to the Wheeling office. IDG meetings were at 8:00 a.m. at the Ohio Valley Medical Center. Then I would see patients in the Wheeling and Moundsville areas. I put almost 50,000 miles on a new Jeep in less than two years because of this schedule. Eventually, more chaplains were hired, and I just saw patients in Monongalia and Preston Counties, which was challenging enough considering the territory's size.

One day I received a referral to see a new hospice patient outside a small town in mountainous Preston County. The patient was an elderly man being cared for by his granddaughter in an old trailer. When I arrived, it was obvious that I was only there because the granddaughter was a Christian and wanted me to visit with her unsaved, stubborn grandfather. He sat there with his arms crossed like he was enduring a root canal during my visit.

When I told him my name, the patient acted surprised as if a bell had just gone off in his mind. "Falkenstine," he said. "Are you any relation to Corky Falkenstine?"

"Yes," I replied (Corky was my uncle's nickname). "That was my uncle, and he died a few years ago." Immediately, the man's countenance brightened.

"Your uncle was a good baseball pitcher, and I was his catcher. We were a team, and we played many baseball games together all over the area." He proceeded to tell me stories of their travels and times together. He told me that he grew up in Newburg, WV. I told him that when I was in college around 1974, I had a job driving a truck making newspaper bundle deliveries throughout Newburg and Preston County. I knew a man by his same last name and recalled where he used to live. I even recalled that his house burned down a few years later. "That was my dad," he said, "and that's the house I grew up in."

Suddenly and providentially, I was now this man's new friend with an inside connection that gave him pleasant memories from his past. It was exciting to see how the Lord used my family connection with my uncle and his experiences from decades earlier to connect with this patient. The Lord used all of this to do an amazing work in this man's life even though all of it was so far from my family's home.

We talked for a while, and I finally brought the conversation around to spiritual things to discover what he believed. It was obvious that he wasn't a Christian, but because I was Corky Falkenstine's nephew, and I had even done my uncle's funeral, he was willing to hear what I had to say. We talked about salvation and what it means to be saved and discussed a scripture that was important to knowing this truth.

Romans 10:9–13 (NLT)

If you confess with your mouth that Jesus is Lord and believe in your heart that God raised him from the dead, you will be saved. For it is by believing in your heart that you are made right with God, and it is by confessing with your mouth that you are saved. As the Scriptures tell us, "Anyone who trusts in him will never be disgraced." Jew and Gentile are the same in this respect. They have the same Lord, who gives generously to all who call on him. For "Everyone who calls on the name of the LORD will be saved."

I could tell this scriptural truth touched his heart, but he needed to "chew on it for a while." I told him I was on call if he needed me. I also told him I would return the following week, and we'd talk more about it then.

Five days later I received a call in the evening from the night RN on-call supervisor. She said the man was declining quickly and was asking for me to come. I made the one-hour drive from Morgantown to rural Preston County to see him, I arrived at about 9:00 p.m. Several family members had gathered at the trailer in support, knowing that he would die soon. When I arrived, his granddaughter got everyone out of the living room, where the patient was now lying in the hospital bed that hospice had provided, and onto the front porch. It was just him and me in the room now.

Though very weak, he awoke when I arrived and responded to me holding his hand. He was on oxygen and was struggling for breath. I had seen this many times before and knew he was "actively dying," as it is called in hospice. He recognized me, so I asked if he had given any thought to what we had last talked about. He nodded. I asked him if he would like to ask Jesus into his heart, so he could go to heaven when he died, and he nodded again. He no longer had the strength to talk and he was in and out of consciousness at times. I prayed with him and for him, asking him to follow along in his heart as best as he could. All I can know on this side of heaven is that I believe he gave his heart to the Lord before dying later that night. The Lord had blessed him and given him one last opportunity to get his heart right with God before dying. This was a hospice chaplain's greatest blessing.

In His providence the Lord was able to use all the complicated details of this whole scenario to His glory and honor. Only God could have weaved together all these events from both our lives to accomplish this. All these relationships from the past had to all come together to allow this man to have his last opportunity to come to Christ.

The Lord only knows whose prayers were answered, prayers that maybe years before from his parents, wife, or granddaughter played a part in the Lord choosing to use me in this way. Only God could use a relationship with my uncle over fifty years earlier and my relationship with this man's father over thirty-five years before to work together to make a difference in this man's life miles away from home.

This was entirely a "God thing." All I had to do was allow Him to work through me to make this difference. God gets all the glory. Again, my job was to just stay attached to the vine and allow God's strength and power to work through me to bear fruit and bring Him glory (John 15:5).

CHAPTER 6

———⋈———

The White House Carpenter

I was always grateful to get to know new patients and hear their life stories. They would share special remembrances and personal experiences that I would have never heard about any other way. As a chaplain, I tried to be a blessing and provide comfort to them; it was usually a mutual blessing to me as we got to know each other.

James "Jimmy" Ray Walters was one of those special individuals who shared his interesting life experiences enthusiastically with me. He told me he was blessed to be able to tell his personal stories and relive them with me, and I was certainly blessed to hear them. Jimmy was a resident at a local nursing home and was admitted to hospice in the spring of 2019. By the time I met him, he was alone and had lost his eyesight. His wife had died, he had no children, and his sister, Carol Rose, was his only close relative. Carol cared deeply for her brother, but she lived in Maryland and wasn't able to come regularly to Morgantown to see him. She had asked that I call her weekly to give her my assessment of how he was doing. Carol gave me permission to share his name as well as his one-of-kind stories with you.

The unique aspect of Jimmy's life and career was that he worked at the White House, in Washington, DC, as the official White House carpenter. He started under Lyndon Johnson and continued through the administrations of Presidents Richard Nixon, Gerald Ford, Jimmy Carter, Ronald Reagan, George Bush, and Bill Clinton before retiring in 1999 because of health issues. His stories were so interesting and colorful, certainly an unwritten part of presidential history. He told me that he dearly loved his job and the excitement involved, and sometimes he hated leaving the White House at the end of the day. He said that his wife was allowed to come to a certain room at the back of the White House when she got off work, just so they would have some time together.

During my weekly visits with Jimmy, he would light up when he heard my voice and was always very respectful of me because of my position as chaplain. He would never call me "Craig." It was always "Chaplain" or "Chaplain Craig." I could see how his respectful and pleasant personality would go over well in dealing with presidents and their family members. He always expressed his appreciation for my visits and prayers for him and wanted to say the Lord's Prayer together. His sister, Carol, had placed many of the pictures he had with presidents and their wives on the walls of his nursing room walls to help generate people's interest and conversation with Jimmy. Most of the pictures had personal notes and were signed by the presidents. I would ask him a question, and he would always launch into a story that offered a behind-the-scenes peek at history.

"Just what does a White House carpenter do?" I asked.

"What didn't I do?" he replied. He said he had a high-security clearance, and because of his years of service, he was counted on to do many sensitive things around the White House. Even after he retired, the Secret Service would check up on him to make sure no one was trying to get classified information out of him.

One of his duties was overseeing staging for White House events. When platforms needed to go up, he was in the middle of it all. He got to meet many famous people as a result. One of his memories was of Elvis Presley coming to sing for President Nixon. While they were setting up, Elvis was talking privately to the president nearby when Elvis pulled out a fancy handgun to show the president. Then the president pulled out a hidden gun he had on him and showed it to Elvis. Jimmy laughed and said he never saw so many Secret Service agents come out of the woodwork, quickly scooping up those guns from them.

He also did a lot of repairs to the presidents' private quarters and fulfilled many personal requests from various presidents. His office was in the basement of the White House near the bowling alley, and Bill Clinton often asked him to bowl with him since he was nearby. George H. W. Bush always asked Jimmy to play horseshoes with him because Jimmy had been a horseshoe champ as a kid. Jimmy said that President Bush never did beat him, and when President Bush lost, he often told Jimmy, jokingly, that he was going to send him to Afghanistan as a result.

When he started working in the White House, Jimmy was downstairs heating up some homemade chili to eat. He turned around, and there stood Lyndon Johnson in Jimmy's office. The president said he had smelled chili and wanted some. Jimmy shared his chili with the president that day.

I asked Jimmy if he was ever in the Oval Office. He said he was there every day for some time because of his security clearance, and they trusted him to be the one to clean it. He got there early and cleaned it before the president arrived in the morning. He always enjoyed waxing the stately floors of the White House, making them look good.

Sometimes I would ask Jimmy different questions, such as: Who was the smartest president? Who was the meanest president? Who was his favorite president? His answers were surprising. He told me that Richard Nixon was the smartest president and that he showed great kindness to the White House staff as well. Nixon made sure all children of White House staff members got the Christmas presents they wanted and that he personally paid for them. As for the meanest president, he said Jimmy Carter was the toughest on staff. His favorite president by far was Ronald Reagan. President Reagan loved a certain kind of jellybeans, and they had dishes of them all over the White House for him. Reagan called him "Big Jim" and was always very personable with him. President Reagan would bring Jimmy wooden toys or puzzles that he wanted him to recreate, so the president could give them as small gifts. He also asked him to make gold picture frames that he could present with a photo gift for special people. The president teased him and called him "Goldfinger" as a result. One time he said Reagan asked him to quickly put together a gold frame with a photo he gave him. He said he would be waiting in the helicopter on the White House lawn for it and to bring it as soon as it was finished. Jimmy quickly put it together, then ran it out to the president, who was waiting in the helicopter. Immediately, the president took off.

I also asked Jimmy what was the scariest time for him while he worked in the White House. He said it was when President

Reagan was shot. Jimmy was in the crowd behind the gunman and the president and saw it all unfold. They created a hospital room on the upper floor of the White House, so President Reagan could be taken care of when he returned to the White House to recuperate.

Another scary time was when a glider plane flew into the White House when President Clinton lived there. Jimmy said he was the first on the scene moments before the Secret Service arrived.

I asked him if he was ever on Air Force One, the president's plane, and he said only once. President Clinton wanted to see a certain baseball game, and the Secret Service were scurrying around trying to find people to be in the audience to help protect the president. They asked Jimmy if he wanted to go to a baseball game. He ended up being part of the motorcade to and from Air Force One and to the game and back. He said it was a lot of fun.

One time Hillary Clinton was trying to figure out where to put pictures on one of the walls in the White House quarters and sat down on the floor trying to decide. "So, I just sat down with her on the floor until she made her decision," Jimmy told me. I asked him what he thought of her. "She was sneaky," he said. I asked if staff knew of President Clinton's "shenanigans" that went on in the White House. "Oh, yes," he replied. "everyone knew."

Because staff practically lived at the White House, they had their own staff cook who provided their meals. He often ate what the president ate. I asked him where the White House got its food. He said people went to supermarkets all over the area and bought the same kind of food everyone else bought. That way no one knew someone was buying food for the White House.

When President Bush was going to be inaugurated, gifts came pouring into the White House, and they put them into a room to hold them. The Bush family told the White House Staff that they couldn't accept the gifts but for the staff members to take any present they liked. Jimmy went in to pick out a gift and saw a big box that had a nice dress inside with matching accessories. He thought it would make a nice gift for his mother, so he took it home with him that night. When he got home, the White House called saying that the dress was Barbara Bush's inaugural dress, which was accidentally put in the room. He needed to bring it back to the White House immediately.

He thought a lot of the Bush family and said they were one of his favorites. He had a good relationship with George and Barbara Bush and the entire family. Even after George Bush lost his re-election and returned to Texas, they invited Jimmy to fly down to visit. He never did take them up on their offer and regretted that he hadn't done so.

When Jimmy's wife died in 2007, long after he had retired, George and Laura Bush (the president at that time) sent him a personal condolence note, which he had framed and hung on his wall.

I asked him about Christmas celebrations at the White House. He said Christmas was a big deal that all the staff had to help with. There would be as many as twenty-nine Christmas trees all over the White House, and everyone had to help decorate them. At Christmas the president and first lady would hold a dress-up Christmas party for staff and their spouses that always resulted in group Christmas photos that were personalized and autographed. Jimmy had many of these on his walls in the nursing home.

As the weeks went on, I could easily tell how Jimmy was doing by his ability to tell me a memory of working at the White House. He loved telling the stories, and it always seemed to cheer him up. As time went on, his stories would get shorter, and he would lose his train of thought. Eventually, he could only acknowledge that I was there, and I would pray for him. He peacefully passed away while I was out of town on July 29, 2019. Jimmy was certainly one of my most memorable patients.

Today, in Beverly, WV, where Jimmy and his wife used to live, there is a display at the heritage museum of some of the photos of Jimmy's time at the White House. The Huttonsville (WV) Hunt Club recently honored Jimmy with a plaque on a bench at Jimmy's favorite deer-hunting spot. A story about it in *The Inter-Mountain* newspaper stated, "He (James) quickly ingratiated himself to the community even while living in Maryland. This became his second home. So much so, he and his wife, June, retired in Beverly, WV."

CHAPTER 7

————————⋈————————

Eyewitness to the Pearl Harbor Attack— God's Hand of Protection

I was always overjoyed to hear stories of people who had lived through well-known historical events. Eyewitness accounts paint a sharp picture of the facts of history that most people only read about. They make things so real and so special, especially, when someone can give a personal testimonial of how God was there to help them through it. So many of these personal stories only last as long as the eyewitness is still alive. If they're not recorded in some way, they're gone.

One of these times was when the husband of one of our hospice patients told me about his experience of being a young Navy sailor aboard one of the ships in Pearl Harbor the day it was bombed on December 7, 1941. I got to know this man (Harry) when his wife was admitted to hospice. Harry was his wife's caregiver and was very dedicated to her care even though he was up in years, was a large man, and had physical and health issues himself. Harry was a pleasant, jovial man and was always appreciative of anything I did for him and loved to talk. He and I became good friends as I regularly visited him and his wife and provided chaplain support to them. They were both strong Christians, so my visits with them were always pleasant and as meaningful to me as I hope they were to them.

One day when I came to visit, Harry told me the story of what had happened to him the night before. He said he drove over to the local convenience store late at night, after his wife was asleep, to pick up some things and fill his gas tank. When he got out of his car at the pumps, he fell and couldn't get up. He said he just prayed, "Lord help me. What am I supposed to do?" Moments later a big young man came around the building and approached Harry, asking if he could help. Harry explained that he couldn't get up because he was so heavy. He said the young man picked him up as if he were a ragdoll and set him on his feet. He even offered to pump his gas for him and take his payment in for him. When he returned and gave everything back to Harry, Harry turned to thank him, but the young man was nowhere in sight. "That man was an angel sent by God," Harry insisted. He said that where that young man came from around the building, there is nothing. The fact that the young man so effortlessly picked him up and then disappeared was more proof.

That led Harry to tell me about another occasion where he felt an angel had protected him from death. Harry was a young man in the Navy during World War II on one of the ships at Pearl Harbor. He described in great detail what a beautiful Sunday morning it was as he and one of his buddies were sitting on the edge of their ship relaxing. They watched the Japanese planes pass over, flying exceptionally low. The planes were so low he said he made eye contact with one of the pilots.

He and his buddy looked at each other as the plane passed and said, "Those aren't American planes." Moments later, in his words, "all hell broke loose."

Harry said he jumped on a machine gun that was mounted on the ship with an integral seat built with it. It was all freshly painted and looked as if it had never been fired. He started firing at the planes as the bombs hit, and the planes fired back. He kept firing until the planes left. When he was done, the machine gun was so hot that the paint had peeled off. He got down from his seat at the machine gun and looked at the wall behind him. He said he immediately realized an angel had protected him from harm because bullet holes filled almost the entire wall. With all those bullet holes there was an obvious outline of where he had been sitting at the gun. He said someone must have been praying for him because the Lord sent an angel to shield him and spared his life that day.

A few months later, I was the first person Harry called when he realized his wife had died early in the morning. Fortunately, I was able to be there within minutes. I stayed with Harry until the nurse came and as the funeral home personnel arrived to take her body. Later, I was able to conduct a memorial service for his wife at a local church. I continued to keep in touch with Harry, and I supported him later in the trials of dealing with selfish adult children and his relocating to a senior facility. Before his death, I was also able to take him to my church for an Easter Service. I did a memorial service for Harry at the seniors' complex where he lived. It was a blessing to have known Harry and his wife and share in their experiences of God's work in their lives.

CHAPTER 8

———◁✕▷———

God's Providence

I want to share another remarkable story of one of my former hospice patients who greatly exhibited God's providence and blessing. The story begins in 2010 when we admitted an elderly former nurse with colon cancer who was discharged from the hospital to go back home. The doctors told her there wasn't much that could be done. Our hospice was called to follow her as the doctors encouraged her to live out the remainder of her life in her modest trailer.

When we admitted the patient, our staff immediately saw a huge emotional and spiritual need, and I was given the referral to see her. During my first visit, the patient was very emotional and not dealing well with her terminal prognosis, still in shock and denial. The patient hadn't been in a church since she was a child. I tried to gently guide her in discussing her thoughts and spiritual beliefs, but she became hysterical and demanded I leave her trailer. She wouldn't even allow me to pray for her. She just threw me out of her home. It was the only time that ever happened in my career. At the time it was very upsetting to me that I couldn't help her. She had such an obvious need for help.

I prayed for the Lord to intervene in her life somehow. Her only active caregiver was a troubled granddaughter. The woman refused to accept what was going on, was in chronic pain, and not receiving enough help from her family. A few days later she revoked hospice services to try to find a doctor who could heal her. Our office didn't hear from her again.

Several months later I received a call late in the afternoon on one of the rare occasions when I was home early. The call was from a nurse from another hospice company who had received a call from a local nursing home. The nursing home was looking for a pastor who could come right away to talk with a dying patient. That particular hospice's chaplain was out of the area, so they called me to see if I could help. No patient name was given, but I told them I would go immediately since I was only two miles away.

When I got to the nursing home and talked with the social worker, she took me to see the patient, who was alone. Her daughter had already left before I got there, saying she couldn't handle it.

When I entered the patient's room, I realized it was the same lady who had thrown me out of her trailer. Her eyes opened wide when she saw me, and she burst into tears. I walked over to her bedside, and she grabbed my hand, holding on to me for dear life for the next forty minutes. I asked her if she remembered me, and she nodded. She told me that she wanted to die but didn't want to die. She was miserable and in pain. She just had been given pain medication, and there was little more that could be done to make her more comfortable.

I began to talk with her but needed to talk loudly into her only good ear, next to the pillow, so she could understand me.

Our discussion came down to the fact that she was afraid to die, but she wanted to die because she was so uncomfortable.

Unlike before, she was now very receptive to anything I had to say and wanted to accept Jesus as her Savior, so she could go to heaven. She prayed with me and gladly said that Jesus was Lord. As she continued to cry from pain, I coached her to remember that phrase and repeat it to herself during those tough times. As I left her room, she was trying to fall asleep and kept saying to herself, "Jesus is Lord. Jesus is Lord..."

Wow. Praise the Lord for his divine appointments and providence. I was able to visit this lady again before her death, and she seemed grateful to see me once again. What a blessing to be a part of God's work of grace, mercy, and providence in her life.

Years later I also visited her daughter and son-in-law. Her son-in-law was dying and being cared for at home, also on hospice. I was honored to do his funeral as well. After her husband died, her daughter came to my widows' retreat at Sandscrest Conference Center in Wheeling, WV. I was blessed to be able to provide and teach at widows' retreats for eighteen years to help ladies cope with the death of their husbands.

CHAPTER 9

———————✂———————

Go Work Your Magic

I received a referral to see a new hospice patient who was living in a nursing home and had just been admitted by our nursing staff. The lady (I'll refer to her as Sally) was in her eighties. She had a reputation among the nursing home staff of being difficult to handle because of her unusual panic-attack outbursts in certain situations. The outbursts always required her to be removed from parties, nursing home events, or other activities and taken to her room. They also required her to be medicated, so she would calm down and go to sleep. She wanted to go to the events but couldn't explain why she had panic attacks. This frustrated Sally, her family, and the nursing home staff. This was another situation where the unbelieving staff said, "Craig, go work your magic." But it wasn't my magic. It was only God, through the power of the Holy Spirit, who could do an amazing work in patient's lives, and that is exactly what He did in Sally's life.

Sally was willing to see me but was extremely cautious and reserved. I began seeing her weekly in the nursing home, as I did many hospice patients in facilities. I was a familiar face to many nursing home residents, who became accustomed to seeing me weekly, greeting and talking with me whether they were a hospice patient of ours or not. This familiarity helped Sally feel safe since she had seen me many times over the years. Now I needed to further earn her trust.

Slowly, Sally began to open up and share with me each week. She seemed to look forward to my visits. When the weather permitted, I would take her outside in her wheelchair and push her around the building. Sometimes I would have someone with me who was interning or a new staff member who was shadowing me, but Sally made it clear she was only talking to me. Over time she began to reveal her history and the story of her life. She always responded well to my prayer for her at the end of each visit and seemed genuinely touched.

One day she revealed to me that she thought God could not take her to heaven because of what she had done in her life. This was a major step forward in our counseling relationship, and I asked if she could tell me why. "What I'm going to tell you, I have never told anyone," she said. She proceeded to tell me difficult stories going back over eighty years into her childhood. Her mother was not in the picture, and her father was not around much, so she was living with her grandmother. She was sexually abused by her uncle as early as four years of age, and she had kept that a secret her entire life. Then she was raped by a boyfriend as a teenager, another secret she kept. When she got married, her husband drank and abused her, and she became a major alcoholic. She had children, one of whom suffered from brain damage as a result of her alcoholism. She carried immense guilt as a result of these experiences.

She still viewed her sexual abuse from a "little girl" perspective as something she was somehow responsible for. It took time for her to allow God to help her see she was the victim. She could no longer view the situation with childlike thinking, believing her abuse was somehow her fault. She believed God was punishing her for it as well. She needed to realize that Jesus died for her and wanted to heal her hurts, even at her age, hurts she had been carrying for her entire life.

Over many months, we did a lot of talking and praying. One day it was obvious to me that the light had come on in her mind. She prayed with me and asked Jesus to forgive her, to come into her life, and to heal her. Jesus "showed up and showed off" in a big way that became obvious to everyone through the absence of further panic attacks. She had a new attitude toward life.

One day, as I was visiting with her, I got a call that I needed to go to the hospital ICU and be with a family where the patient was on a ventilator that was about to be removed, so the patient could die. Sally understood that I needed to leave. "Craig," she said before I left, "will you be with me when I die?" Oh my. "All of that is in God's hands," I replied, "but we can ask Him to allow that to happen." We prayed together that day and asked God if He would honor her request.

One Sunday afternoon I got a call that Sally was declining toward death, and she and her family wanted me to come and pray with her. When I arrived at the nursing home, I prayed with her. This seemed to give her some peace. I stayed with her for a while. Her vital signs remained stable, and she was sleeping, but she was not showing any signs that it was her time to be with the Lord. I went home, but the next morning I went back to the nursing home to be with her. I told her that I was there with her and prayed that the Lord would take her peacefully to be with Him soon.

Within the hour, she died peacefully while I was with her, along with some of her family. The Lord had answered her prayers and glorified Himself in the process.

CHAPTER 10

————————⋉————————

My Grandfather's Cross

I was at the hospice booth along with other staff at the 2015 Mon General Health Fair in the Morgantown Mall greeting the crowd as they walked by. Bud Goodwin, a man in his eighties whom I hadn't seen in years, came by. I had met Bud and his wife Helen several years earlier when I performed the funeral service for my dad's cousin's wife, Ruth Falkenstine, at Sugar Valley United Methodist Church in Bruceton Mills, WV.

Helen came up to me and introduced herself and asked if I was the grandson of J. C. McGee and the son of Clarice. I said that I was, and she proceeded to tell me an amazing story that I want to share.

Helen's older sister and my mother, Clarice, were childhood friends and would often play with each other when they were young girls. Helen said her mother was a single parent who worked. When Helen's much older sister went somewhere, Helen had to be the tagalong, bratty little sister who went as well. She said she was always cramping her sister's style whenever she went along.

One day she and her older sister were over at my grandparents' house playing with my mother. Helen said she was being particularly bratty that day and annoying the two older girls. So, my Grandpa McGee took her downstairs into the garage/basement of the house, and my grandfather proceeded to tell her stories. He had been a teacher when he was younger, teaching in a one-room schoolhouse.

As he told her stories, he took two pennies out of his pocket, placed them on an anvil, and then started to pound on them. He pounded and pounded, moving them around and slowly started to fashion the two pennies together in the shape of a cross. She was spellbound as she watched the transformation. When he was finished, my grandfather gave her the cross. She said it became incredibly special to her, and she carried it with her always.

Right there in the church, she took out her change purse and there among her coins was that cross made by grandfather, perhaps seventy to seventy-five years before. She said she had carried that cross in her purse her entire life. I was thrilled to hear that story and to see the cross. It was exciting to know that my grandfather had done something so thoughtful and special for a little girl that it lasted a lifetime and had made a difference in her life. I boldly expressed an interest in having that cross, but she told me that it was too special to her, and she wouldn't part with it.

The following year, on May 25, 2008, I was asked to do the funeral for Maxine Falkenstine Darby, who was my dad's first cousin and was also a hospice patient of ours. We had grown close during her illness, and I was honored that she wanted me to do her service.

Following the funeral at Sugar Valley UMC, in the church basement, the church ladies had gone all out for a wonderful lunch, as they always did. It was there that I saw Bud and Helen Goodwin again. They knew they would see me, and Bud was tickled to give me a gift. He had brought me a beautiful hand-lathed wooden vase with a hand-carved stem and a lid that he had made himself. In the back of my mind, I was thinking maybe they felt guilty for not giving me the cross, but I appreciated their thoughtfulness, and I still treasure that gift. Helen died on March 26, 2010, but I was unable to make it to the funeral home to see Bud.

I was glad to see Bud again at the 2015 Health Fair when he stopped to talk with me at our booth. He had a stroke and had some difficulty talking, and he walked with a limp. I told him that I still had the vase he had made me, sitting on the window ledge of my home office. He beamed as I told him. I also said I was so thrilled to know the story that Helen had told me about the cross that my grandfather made her. He came back to me later and asked where my office was, and I gave him my business card.

The following Monday morning, I was getting into my car to go to the nursing home when Bud drove up in his car, waving to me. He gave me a piece of paper with something wrapped inside. It was the cross my grandfather had made.

How special it was to have that cross, made by my grandfather almost eighty years before, which had meant so much to Helen throughout her life. The interesting thing was that he gave me that cross on the anniversary of my mother's death, March 2. "The gift of the cross keeps on giving in more ways than one."

CHAPTER 11

---⋈---

God Using Hometown Connections

I f there is anything we don't understand, it's the mysterious ways in which God weaves the lives of others in and out of our lives over the years. This includes the purposes we play in their lives and the influences they have on ours, even if we don't realize or appreciate those influences until years later.

Many of the hospice patients I dealt with in Morgantown were people I had known in one way or another over the years. Growing up and still living in the same town as an adult has many advantages that the Lord continually used in my role as a chaplain, though sometimes having a prior relationship with a patient and family made it emotionally difficult to deal with the situation. With a family I did not know, I was able to maintain a healthy professional separation in my heart. I was stepping into their lives to help, always knowing that someday the patient would be dying. I thought the Lord had placed me in their lives to help, and I was blessed to get to know them. I would never have met them any other way. It seems I could deal with my grief better when I lost such patients. But they were still hospice patients whom I had come to know and love, so I still mourned them in some way.

Many times when I did a funeral for a hospice patient, it seemed as therapeutic for me as I hoped it was for the family. It allowed me to work through my own emotions and deal with my grief in a healthy manner.

With a patient and family that I knew and had a prior relationship with, I would grieve the loss and feel some of the pain as well. It was always emotionally draining. An example was when a friend from church was dying after a long battle with cancer. It was hard to see him so thin, frail, and declining. It was emotionally draining to try to support my friends. In this case, I was able to come back to the house with the nurse as the man was dying. When he took his last breath, I was holding his hand. In the midst of all the stress, my own heart went into atrial fibrillation (irregular heart rhythm). This had occurred several times over the years, and I knew how to safely deal with it, but no one else knew what was happening to me. It became one of the hazards of dealing with death and dying.

Many of my high school friends had parents who became hospice patients over the years. Knowing the family background made it easier to provide meaningful support and conversation with them. I was able to be a support when their kids lived out of town and couldn't always be with them. In many ways it was therapeutic to me because I was able to support these parents in ways that I was unable to support my own.

However, sometimes those blessings of relationships from the past created emotionally stressful hospice situations. I was glad to be there to help, but it was emotionally stressful for me to deal with another loss. I had to follow my own advice on grieving effectively and not allowing the grief to accumulate on the job.

I experienced many such situations over the years with special people whom I loved. Examples include two incredibly special ladies where it was gratifying to visit and provide chaplain support to them at the end of their lives. Both of these ladies were like second moms to me at different times in my life. It was very meaningful for me to be part of their lives when they needed end-of-life support.

One of these special ladies was Ann Wiley. She was the youngest of all the neighborhood moms growing up and had a lot of time and energy for us as kids. Her oldest son, John, and I were the same age. Four of us were the same age in the neighborhood, and we did many things together growing up. Mrs. Wiley would pile all of us in her blue Ford station wagon and chauffeur us all over the place. She even taught us how to water ski at Cheat Lake where we did a lot of summer boating in those days. She also picked us up and took us to school almost every morning before we learned to drive.

The first time my parents left me home alone for a trip to Baltimore, I was fifteen and still in school. I thought I was really on my own. My parents left Thursday night, so I thought Friday would be a good day to sleep in, skip school, and make a long weekend for myself. Well, at 9:00 a.m. the phone rang. It was Mrs. Wiley saying she noticed I didn't make it to school on time. She said would be by to take me to school in a few minutes. It was a parent conspiracy.

I had the chance to visit her when she was a hospice patient and provide support to John, who did a great job of providing care for her. I was able to tell her how much I appreciated her and what she meant to me growing up and during my junior and senior high school years. I especially appreciated the support she gave me when my father died. It was a meaningful time for us both. She also appreciated my being there to pray for her, and I was blessed to do so.

Another special second mom to me was Lois Wiles. I always had a good relationship with Floyd and Lois because their son, Bill, was, and still is, one of my closest friends. Our friendship goes back to the 1960s when we met at church. From the time my mom died, Lois seemed to adopt me as another son. I spent my first Christmas without my mom with the Wiles family.

My mom had dearly loved Bill. She knew what few vegetables he would eat and would fix them for him when she invited him to eat at our house. I think I could have told mom that I was robbing a bank, and it would have been OK if I was doing it with Bill.

After my grandmother died, my family always spent Christmas Eve with the Wiles family, having dinner before going to the candlelight service at church. One time Bill, who now lived in California, asked me to take Lois out and help her buy a new car. It was a special time for us.

Now Lois had become a hospice patient, though she was able to stay at home with caregivers as well as great care from her other son, Bob. During this time, Floyd died suddenly. I continued to visit Lois every Tuesday, providing support until she died. She always appreciated me praying for her and encouraging her during those difficult times. I was honored when I was listed in her obituary as her "adopted" son.

CHAPTER 12

∞

Things Don't Always Go as We Hope

The Lord often used my special hometown relationships in positive ways, but sometimes, they didn't go as I hoped or expected. One of these relationships goes back to my days as a paperboy. One of the people I delivered newspapers to was a lady who was a teacher (I'll call her Jane). I collected money for the newspapers every Saturday. Over time, I developed a relationship with her and her elderly mother.

A few years later when I became the first WVU student to be elected to Morgantown City Council, she called to say she wanted me to get the city to put up a stop sign in a certain place (I did so). Later, she wanted me to help get the neighbor's property fixed up (I couldn't).

Over thirty five years later, decades of smoking had taken a toll on her health. Jane had severe COPD (chronic obstructive pulmonary disease) and was admitted to hospice. Her mother and husband had died, and her children lived out of town. She still lived alone in the same house and had a part-time caregiver. She was on her oxygen concentrator 24/7 with tubing long enough to go to every room in her house.

Jane was thrilled to see me again, and I regularly came to visit as her chaplain. She loved to talk but often had to stop talking because she couldn't catch her breath. She would be fighting for air as she tried to talk and would say, "You talk; I can't talk anymore." She was very opinionated and set in her ways. She would ask me what I thought about God, listen to what I had to say, then tell me she didn't believe it that way. Although she used to attend a Methodist church and believed in God, she didn't believe in the Bible and the necessity to accept Jesus as her savior. She would tell me, "I was okay before I was born, so I'll be okay after I die."

Over the course of two years, she became attached to me, and she loved to have me come as often as I could. She felt comfortable with me, and I provided a great deal of socialization and emotional support for her. She was an artist and even gave me a watercolor painting. She would always allow me to pray for her but was unwilling to consider any biblical viewpoints. I continued to ask the Lord to draw her to himself and bring her to a saving knowledge of Jesus before she died.

After a dramatic decline in her health, I received word that she wanted to go to the hospital rather than stay at home on hospice. When I arrived at the hospital, she was alone and panicking because she was so short of breath. Many times COPD patients are anxious because they have trouble breathing, but they are so focused on breathing that their anxiety actually makes it worse. I had seen this happen with her before. I knew if I distracted her, so she could think about something else, she would relax, and her breathing would become easier.

The hospital staff came and tried to give her morphine to help her breathe easier. Jane saw me and waved for me to come and hold her hand. She was extremely glad to have me there with her. She held my hand in a death grip. After trying to coordinate her care with staff, I asked if I could pray for her to give her comfort. She closed her eyes, and I could see the fear on her face as she squeezed my hand. As I was praying for her, suddenly, her grip loosened. That was it. The door was now closed on her ability to make any decision to accept Christ. Her choice was now final, one way or the other.

In a way I felt I had failed her because, to my knowledge, she had never come to accept Christ and his teachings. I needed to process this ending of our relationship and my efforts as a chaplain to make a difference in her life. Had I failed? Was there something I could have changed? I needed to process my feelings. Sometimes I viewed other such situations as failures, but were they really failures on my part?

With some patients I quickly realized the door was already closed for them to be able to have any relationship with the Lord. Dementia, a coma, disease process, and medication all prevented me from making any meaningful difference. There was nothing I could do to change the situation or to help change a heart. I could only pray and provide support for the involved people, caregivers, or family members. I made a sincere effort to receive the Lord's strength to help make a positive difference in their lives.

But I realized I could only be responsible for doing my part. I could not make a decision for anyone else. I had to acknowledge that individuals make their own decisions and must accept the consequences. Each of us can choose to believe a lie or the truth of Scripture or even believe that Scripture is God's Word for us. An individual's choice of salvation is that person's choice alone and is between them and God. But it was always a letdown for me as a chaplain when my hopes and desires for a patient or family weren't realized to my expectations. But, right or wrong, it's still each patient's choice that only they are responsible for.

CHAPTER 13

---⌒×⌒---

Consequences Follow Poor Choices

As I mentioned before, we can choose our choices, but we can't choose the consequences that follow our choices. When I visited hospice patients, our hospice staff would always try to make sure patients were safe and in a safe environment. Patient safety is always a priority, but it comes with personal responsibility. People must do their part to be safe.

One time I visited a lady who lived alone, was on oxygen, but was a heavy smoker. Being a smoker is always a red flag for hospice staff, and everyone tries their best to educate and impress upon patients not to let oxygen and fire mix. I've seen what one hospice patient's face looked like when they forgot to take off his nasal cannula (the part of the oxygen tubing that goes into the patient's nose) before lighting a cigarette. The man's face looked like raw hamburger with burns all over it, even inside his nose. He was fortunate that's all that happened to him.

The woman I was visiting, who was younger than me, liked to smoke in bed. I warned her about the dangers of smoking in bed as well as smoking around oxygen. Smoking is likely what caused her terminal illness to begin with. She casually told me she was always careful and took her oxygen cannula off and placed it on her bed when she smoked. She even demonstrated how she did it, which didn't make me feel any better.

Unfortunately, one time she took her oxygen off and placed it on her bed, then put her lit cigarette next to the oxygen tubing. It caught her bed on fire, which caught the entire house on fire.

When the fireman arrived, they found her on the floor next to her bed with very severe burns—she must have been able to roll herself out of bed. When I saw her the next day, all they could do was try to keep her comfortable until she died. Her nylon nightgown had melted into her skin and couldn't be taken off. Most of her hair was melted or burned to her head. The smell of burned flesh is terrible. Even though she was very sedated, she moaned continually. She seemed to acknowledge me, and all I could do was pray for her.

Unfortunately, her son was in jail. The authorities gave him the choice of coming to the hospital to see his mother while she was still alive or going to her funeral. He couldn't do both. I was in her hospital room when the guards brought him in wearing his orange prison jumpsuit along with handcuffs and ankle chains. They let me be in the room with him on one side of the bed and me on the other. The guards stood in the doorway and watched us. The poor kid could only cry as I tried to comfort him. He hadn't seen his mother since his trial and didn't know she was so sick, let alone the consequences of the fire. I think she sensed he was there by the way she reacted. I did her funeral a few days later.

Several years later, I tried to call another hospice patient to tell her I was coming to see her. She lived in a very rural area. However, all I got on the phone was a strange ringing noise. I decided to go ahead and make the hour-long trip anyway since I knew she was bedridden.

I was shocked and horrified when I arrived at her home and found it burned to the ground with smoke still rising from the ashes. Later, I discovered that a few hours before, she had been smoking in bed with her oxygen tube lying beside her. The fire killed her and the little dog that slept with her, and a family member was seriously burned trying to get into the room to attempt to save her. The entire house burned to the ground before the fire department could arrive.

During my last visit to her, I had warned her once again that she shouldn't smoke with the oxygen around. I even told her the awful story of the other lady who died as a result of smoking in bed. This patient also told me, "I'm always careful."

Thoughts About
Patient Care:

CHAPTER 14

———————◁×▷———————

What Would They Have Wanted Me to Do?

"I wish they would have told me what they wanted." This is the agony and the reality for some hospice families trying to guess what type of medical decisions to make for a comatose family member. Many families need to make a critical medical decision when the patients can no longer express their own wishes or desires. It's emotionally difficult for families to make such hard discussions about keeping someone alive, often artificially. These situations resulted in great agony and guilt for families. Tough questions that should be discussed by families in advance are:

- When your heart stops or when you quit breathing after a long illness, what is to be done? Would you like to be a DNR (do not resuscitate), so you can die in peace without the EMS squad coming to do CPR (cardiopulmonary resuscitation)? CPR is not a pretty picture for any family member to watch and has limited results. Doing CPR often means being put on a ventilator to keep you alive if you are resuscitated.

- Do you want a feeding tube when they can no longer feed yourself? If so, for how long?
- Do you want IV hydration when you can no longer drink. If so, for how long?
- Do you want to be put on a ventilator to be kept alive? If so, for how long?
- Who do you want to make your medical decisions when you no longer can? (Can this family member handle the pressure put on him or her?)
- What kind of treatments do you want or don't want to be kept alive?

It's a matter of developing a plan ahead of time. Then, if or when a medical crisis hits, your family will be able to refer to it. It's a loving thing for anyone to have a plan in place for their family.

My son, Evan, was part of the original effort to put advanced directives into a West Virginia statewide computer directory to share individuals' medical wishes. The West Virginia Center for End-of-Life Care provides help with all advance-care planning needs. This nationally recognized center provides coordination, education, and resources to ensure patients' wishes are known and respected.

Booklets and websites are available to help social workers support patients and families meet this need. Knowing what the patient's wishes are helps take the stress (and guilt) off families. A great deal of information is required to make an informed medical decision. It usually takes someone else, such as a social worker, to help walk people through these serious issues.

With each hospice admission, a social worker, nurse, or chaplain will ask whether the patient wants to be a DNR or a full code (CPR). An answer to that question by either the patient or family is always an indicator of whether they have given much thought to end-of-life issues. Some patients are very decisive in giving a DNR order and have no problem saying, "When it's my time to go, just let me go." I often saw patients with a faith background who were confident about where their soul was going when they died, so they had peace in their decision.

When a patient or family wanted CPR, even though the patient had a debilitating disease, it always required much more discussion. Many times it was a spiritual issue of being afraid to die. Patients didn't know where they were going when they died, so they wanted to be kept alive no matter what. Our staff provided education about each end-of-life choice and its consequences, but, right or wrong, it still is the patient's right to choose the type of care they want.

CHAPTER 15

————⚬————

Curative or Palliative Care

S ometimes patients who have a serious life-threatening illness need to decide if it's time to move from curative to
palliative care.

Curative care focuses on seeking a cure whatever those
treatments might involve. Many people choose to be treated
until they die and accept all the side effects that go along with
that choice. However, some patients must decide whether
they want a quality of life without treatment side effects or
possible quantity of life while tolerating various side effects.
There are also times when patients don't get to choose.

Palliative care provides a holistic approach to care, focusing
on physical, emotional, social, and spiritual issues. It is the
transition to no longer seeking a cure or realizing that there is
no cure. It doesn't mean giving up; rather, the patient's desire
is to be made as comfortable as possible as they conclude their
life. Hospice care comes at the end of this time and is often
described as striving to give the best quality of life until life's
end. Curative treatments, like chemotherapy for cancer, often

have side effects that affect the quality of life and don't necessarily provide quantity of life.

This discussion needs to include family members and the patient's physicians. It's a matter of looking at the patient's prognosis and the benefits and intent of treatment. Many factors need to be considered, so patients and their families are able to make an informed decision. Many times it comes down to whether patients want to be treated until they die.

CHAPTER 16

———————⋈———————

Hospice Care for Terminally Ill Patients

When a patient is admitted to hospice, a doctor certifies that they believe the patient, with a terminal diagnosis has six months or less to live. That doesn't mean the patient will necessarily die within six months. It's merely the physician's best judgment at the time, a judgment that is necessary to begin the hospice process. This hospice decision needs to be recertified at ninety- or sixty-day intervals to ensure the patient is still appropriate for the hospice benefit. In the United States, one hundred percent of the cost for the hospice benefit is covered for Medicare-age individuals. We often had patients who were in hospice care for years because their health went through waves of decline and improvement. Sometime after admission they were discharged because they actually improved with hospice care and then were readmitted when they declined. I remember one patient whom we didn't think was going to last a week. She was in extremely poor condition, bedbound, and looked as if she could die any minute. She was fortunate to have had a dedicated daughter, a retired nurse, who took wonderful care of her. That woman lasted over seven years, going on and off hospice support several times. Another lady was on and off hospice many times over the years as well and lived to be 110. As a hospice chaplain, I always say, "Only the Lord knows the number of days ordained for us" (Psalm 139:16).

Hospice never includes euthanasia. The hospice benefit provides medications to help ensure patients' comfort, but nothing is given to hasten death. The goal of hospice is to provide the best quality of life until life's end. Many families and patients struggle with experiencing extreme physical decline and pain as a patient's health spirals down. This is understandable. Their quality of life seems to be visibly disappearing before their family's very eyes.

Patients and family members often say, "Wouldn't it be better if they just died or were put out of their misery?" Unfortunately, this line of reasoning is usually taken from a secular viewpoint where people have not allowed God to be part of their lives. Some people compare this thinking to animal caregivers who love their pets and don't want to see them suffer. They see euthanizing their animals as a kindness (which it is). People who lack faith think what is good for animals should work for people as well. God's perspective makes all the difference and is the necessary basis for our thinking about life and death. The following passage in Psalm 139 reminds us that God is our Creator, and he is in charge of and knows our days.

Psalm 139:13–17 (NLT)

You made all the delicate, inner parts of my body and knit me together in my mother's womb.

Thank you for making me so wonderfully complex. Your workmanship is marvelous—how well I know it.

You watched me as I was being formed in utter seclusion, as I was woven together in the dark of the womb.

You saw me before I was born. Every day of my life was recorded in your book. Every moment was laid out before a single day had passed.

How precious are your thoughts about me, O God. They cannot be numbered.

Every human being has a soul and a body made by God's watchful eye which is always on them, whether they realize it or not. Our beloved pets and animals who are loved and then euthanized have no souls. Our human soul is the only thing we take with us to heaven.

I've had many discussions with hospice patients and caregivers who felt that God had abandoned them because they were in such terrible physical condition. Patients don't like being a burden to their families, and they see no good in their end-of-life situation. They wish it was just over. But there's a bigger picture to all of this. Many patients or family members have asked me to pray that the Lord would just let them die. Many times the Lord has quickly answered such prayers, but God is still on the throne and in charge, so his perspective must be considered.

CHAPTER 17

—✕—

What Good Could Possibly Come Out of This?

The hospice experience for God-believing patients is also the realization that what they are going through now is God working for His good in the hearts of caregivers and the entire family. It's not a wasted situation, struggle, or experience. God is using all of it. He is using the patient as a teacher. I have encouraged and tried to help patients realize they are modeling a behavior for their entire family. They are showing the younger generations what it looks like to trust the Lord as they die as Christians, knowing that the best is yet to come. It's important for patients who have always been "givers" in their families to allow their family to give to them now and be the loving caregivers.

It's also important for one generation to teach the next "how it's done," demonstrating that the hospice caregiving situation is what a loving family does to provide care for the older generation for the remainder of their days. Indeed, it is the fulfilment of the biblical command to "honor your father and mother." As the younger generation sees how their parents are taking care of their grandparents, hopefully, when it's the next generation's turn at this life cycle, they know how it's done because they have already observed it firsthand. They have witnessed the personal sacrifices made to lovingly provide care to all members of the family. Family taking care of family is always what's important and beneficial.

Ideally, family members and caregivers see an authentic Christian, someone with a personal relationship with Jesus, who has peace and grace (provided by the Lord) in knowing where they are going when they die. They all learn firsthand what a real believer in Christ does in trusting the Lord for the remainder of their days. Believers in Christ are confident that this life is not all there is. The best (heaven) is yet to come for all of us who trust in Jesus. I can attest that the Lord takes care of His own. God's grace is indeed sufficient.

2 Corinthians 12:9 (ESV)

But he said to me, "My grace is sufficient for you, for my power is made perfect in weakness." Therefore, I will boast all the more gladly of my weaknesses, so that the power of Christ may rest upon me.

CHAPTER 18

———————⌒✕⌒———————

Meaningful Conversations with Hospice Patients

Many families struggle with knowing what they should say to someone they love who is dying or how to have a meaningful conversation with a hospice patient. Trying to start a serious discussion time is usually difficult, uncomfortable, and awkward. However, you can only talk about the weather for so long before you run out of words. Patients get tired of people asking them how they feel today. However, some people don't know what to say or do, so they don't say or do anything.

Hospice patients who are talking with family, with people they love, want to have a short, meaningful conversation. Families need to realize that meaningful, clear-headed, conversations with hospice patients can be a rare and short-lived gift. Treasure these times. Some patients, because of the disease process or even their personalities, may not always be able to articulate their love and appreciation to their family members. But families should always feel free to express their love and appreciation for the patient. Prayers said aloud for the patient are also meaningful and an encouragement. It's great if you are able to talk to the patient when he or she can respond, but it's still important to express your feelings to the patient even if he or she is comatose or unresponsive. This expression becomes an important beginning step for the family to work through their anticipatory grief.

Anticipatory grief often begins without caregivers and family realizing what's happening. Family members or caregivers begin to anticipate that the person is going to die soon and begin to grieve the loss. This is a normal and often a healthy response to this sad time. Such people aren't in denial of what's happening; they are merely beginning the grieving process. Many widows have told me that as their husbands were declining, they began to grieve their loss little by little over time as certain elements of their relationship began to fade. They processed and worked through their grief during this hospice process and the patient's decline, feeling that they were in a better place in their bereavement journey for having done so. This process is certainly enhanced when a chaplain, social worker, nurse, pastor, or even a close friend listens to and supports them during this time.

Meaningful conversations to have with hospice patients include family members or friends telling them what they loved most about them and reliving stories. You can also share what you are thankful to God about regarding them or tell the patient what you will miss the most about them. You can also tell them something you will always remember about your relationship or recall what you learned from the patient. Such conversations, even if they are one-sided or highly emotional, are important. It's great if the patient is conscious and can hear you, but it is equally important for you to share with the unconscious patient as an expression of your love and to begin to express your grief. Many professionals feel that hearing is the last sense to leave and that patients can still hear even though they can't respond. This meaningful communication helps facilitate a more meaningful hospice experience for patients and families as they begin the grief journey. Many find this to be an incredibly special spiritual experience for everyone involved.

CHAPTER 19

———————∝———————

Children's Involvement Is Important

C hildren should not be excluded from caring for terminally ill loved ones. It's important to clearly educate and communicate with kids what is happening. Allow children to help in whatever they can, and don't try to shield or protect them from this part of life. Children's participation in caring for loved family members is difficult but is beneficial for children and will help them mature into loving, caring adults.

Children learn from these important life lessons, even though for adults it's emotional and difficult. These important family events become valuable, life-shaping motivators that help guide children into becoming responsible adults who desire to make a difference in their world. It is all part of God's plan as He works in individual lives and circumstances. Remember that illness, death, and dying are a major part of life for everyone and cannot be avoided. It is important that adults fully explain what is going on to help prevent fear in their children.

If you were to do a survey of hospital professionals who are willing to undergo years of education to prepare them to help people, you would probably find individuals who have had a difficult personal experience that helped shape their life's work. They are now motivated to make a positive difference for others.

Grief/Bereavement Recovery:

CHAPTER 20

You Don't Get Over Your Grief

No matter your occupation or place in life, grief can affect you in many ways. Grief is attached to any kind of loss. Loss and grief go hand in hand. Whether it's a primary loss or a secondary loss, grief impacts our lives. A primary loss is the death of a loved one. A secondary loss isn't as obvious. Sometimes we don't fully recognize grief when it slips in the back door and subconsciously complicates our lives. We often don't recognize grief because we don't realize what we are going through is a loss. Any loss has grief attached to it, and we must deal with our grief if we want to improve our emotional state. Examples of grief sneaking up on us include graduating from school and leaving behind the friends we socialized with every day, being laid off from a job and losing the identity that the job provided, amputation of a limb and the loss of a normal life, miscarriage of a baby and the dream of raising a child, loss of reputation because of a lie or an arrest, loss of self-esteem, loss of a dream, loss of a marriage...The list is endless, but you see the point. Everyone should be aware of grief and do a self-examination of the losses in their lives and the impacts they have had on their frame of mind.

I have seen the grief caused by death change an individual's personality, some for good and some for bad. It all depends on the level of bereavement support an individual receives or is willing to receive. People in culture generally have a hard time correctly supporting and dealing with death and bereavement. A company may offer three days of bereavement leave, and then employees are supposed to go back to normal life. Unfortunately, many people don't know how to respond to bereaved individuals, so they don't say or do anything to help. Thankfully, educating individuals on grief support has come a long way in the fifty years since I needed grief support as a child. It still needs to be addressed as we move forward in the twenty-first century.

For the past thirty-five years, I have been on a quest to provide bereavement support to as many people as possible. I realize what bereavement support could have done for me as a child and certainly what it could have done to support my mother as a young widow. My development of a widow's retreat grew out of seeing my mother struggle through that time. It put me on a track to try to help make a difference in the world of bereavement support.

After my mother died in 1982, I helped start a bereavement support group at church while my wife (my girlfriend at the time) supported those who were divorced. All we did was get like-minded people together to share and help each other. It was called LADD ministries (Life After Death & Divorce). It allowed me to do church bereavement support before I became involved with hospice. Eventually, I became one of the founders of a non-profit organization called the West Virginia Family Grief Center, Inc. (WVFGC). I'm still president of the board of directors. WVFGC helps children and families cope with the death of a loved one. Rather than therapy, the center provides peer support, education, and outreach. Our mission is to provide caring support to grieving children in a safe and comfortable environment. We also have a community bereavement support group for anyone who is dealing with the death of a loved one. During the pandemic, we moved our bereavement support groups online using Zoom, which allowed us to continue to meet a need despite the isolation. Learning to be flexible to meet the current need is important.

Peer support remains an important element of bereavement. As a boy, I discovered the importance of peer support without even knowing what it was. As a boy who lost his dad and was dealing with a grieving mother, it was a friend (peer) who provided the greatest support. That friend's father died not long before mine under the same set of circumstances. Without realizing it, we supported each other because we understood each other's unique grief pain. Our other friends didn't have a clue about grief and the effects it had on the two of us and our families. I remember commenting about the first anniversary of my dad's death to another friend. "I thought you'd be over that (grief) by now," my friend replied. I remember how hurtful that was at the time as I just kept my mouth shut. That friend didn't have a clue about death and grief. He didn't lose his dad and mom until he was an adult. I don't think he meant for it to be hurtful. His words were spoken out of ignorance.

Well-meaning people today still say things out of ignorance; "You need to get over your grief." They think they are being helpful by pushing or even bullying people into dealing or moving on with their grief, as if that were somehow helpful.

In reality, we don't ever get over our grief—and we don't want to. The only way we would totally "get over" our grief would be if someone erased our memories of that person, and we certainly wouldn't want that. This comment surprises some people though. Usually, thoughtless comments are made by people who have never experienced a primary death or a major grief event firsthand. Unfortunately, this lesson is sometimes only taught by the school of hard knocks.

Your bereavement goal should be to work through your grief or to grow through your grief, to be able to turn your pain into a purpose." You don't want to forget the person who died and their influence and place in your life. You want their memories to continue to live in your heart and forever be a part of you. You just want the pain to go away. But you must learn to move toward the grief pain and work through it. You can't, and you shouldn't try to avoid the pain or medicate it away. Work through it on the "head" and "heart" levels. If you genuinely want to heal from your grief pain, you must do the hard work of mourning. Your goal is to grow as a person and develop a new purpose in life as a result of having mourned.

So, what are we to do? Jesus himself told us the answer to this question. Even though the following verse has more than one application, its application to grief is pertinent.

Matthew 5:4 (ESV)

Blessed are those who mourn, for they shall be comforted.

Mourning Is Crucial

If we want God's comfort, we must do the work of mourning. Grief is the emotion on the inside but mourning and grieving are the actions we must take to express those feelings. It's like opening a dark closet door and letting the light come in. It reminds me of one definition of darkness: the absence of light. We can't wait for it to happen on its own. We must acknowledge our grief and work through it if we are to grow. It's a difficult and often time-consuming process. Grief can be tiring, overwhelming, and debilitating. Some people seem to work through it quickly while others struggle as it takes longer than anyone wants. Your personality and all the grief struggles involved in it make it an incredibly unique experience for each person.

Dealing with grief is not a do-it-yourself project. You need the help of friends and often professionals. Grief education encourages people to open the doors of their "grief closets." Bereavement support groups are also valuable tools to help work through grief issues and receive support as people learn to grow through their grief.

Over the Lips or Through the Fingertips

I helped start and taught at a widows retreat called Healing Hearts Retreat for Widows for eighteen years. The retreat was offered at no cost to the wives of our hospice patients. We took the ladies who were willing to go to an old mansion with a beautiful country setting. The mansion had been willed to a church denomination and was turned into a small conference center/resort. It was a delightful place. The widows stayed in the old mansion for two days, and a chef fixed them fabulous meals, which we shared in the old dining room. The groups were always small, around ten women or less. We did some fun craft therapy that helped the ladies to get to know each other and tell their stories of loss. I also provided a lot of teaching using a curriculum I developed over the years. I taught them how to cope and guided them through learning to work through their grief issues. They learned the importance of doing the hard work of mourning.

I always taught bereavement groups the vital need to express their grief. I emphasized the need to move their grief from inside of themselves to the outside. Expressing grief pain is usually done in one of two main ways. I picked up a saying along the way that uniquely expresses this idea, and I repeated it often: "Over the lips or through the fingertips." It easily reminds people of two important ways to express their grief pain. The goal is to be able to mourn effectively and enable them to grow toward healing. In the following two sections, I explain what this expression means.

Over the Lips

Being able to express or talk about your grief is particularly important. Of course, as a believer in Jesus, the first person to talk to is God. You need to talk, pray, and cry out regarding your grief to the Lord in great detail. You need to express your pain and emotions fully to Him. You can even express your anger that your loved one has died. You may never get answers to your questions of "why" it happened, but crying out to God is greatly beneficial in your walk with the Lord. Just as you avoid someone and have a "cold" relationship with them when you are mad or haven't forgiven them, you can inadvertently give God the cold shoulder. Your trust in the Lord may become damaged as a result, and you accidentally build a wall between you and Him when you fail to cry out to the Lord. The Bible contains many psalms that tell us to cry out to God for help. Remember that Jesus is referred to as the "light of the world" and is the perfect one to be your light in the dark closet of grief.

Psalm 3:4 (NLT)

I cried out to the LORD, and he answered me from his holy mountain.

Psalm 34:17–18 (NLT)

The LORD hears his people when they call to him for help. He rescues them from all their troubles.
The LORD is close to the brokenhearted; he rescues those whose spirits are crushed.

Psalm 86:3–7 (NLT)

Be merciful to me, O Lord, for I am calling on you constantly.
Give me happiness, O Lord, for I give myself to you.
O Lord, you are so good, so ready to forgive, so full of unfailing love for all who ask for your help.
Listen closely to my prayer, O LORD; hear my urgent cry.
I will call to you whenever I'm in trouble, and you will answer me.

Another "over the lips" activity is talking to someone about your grief. Joining a bereavement support group is a good place to start. It allows you to share your burdens with other like-minded individuals who understand and identify with your grief-induced pain. The other group members will be incredibly supportive and encouraging to you because they have walked in your shoes. The greatest healing or growth for any bereaved person occurs when they can provide words of encouragement to someone else who is new to the group and recently lost a loved one. This positive growth is an important step in the healing process. A passage in 2 Corinthians addresses this.

2 Corinthians 1:3–5 (NLT)

All praise to God, the Father of our Lord Jesus Christ. God is our merciful Father and the source of all comfort. He comforts us in all our troubles so that we can comfort others. When they are troubled, we will be able to give them the same comfort God has given us. For the more we suffer for Christ, the more God will shower us with his comfort through Christ.

God comforts us not to make us comfortable but to make us comforters. We become credible, living proof that life continues after intense grief, that we can indeed become strong again and emerge from our grief as more mature individuals with a new ability to help others who are hurting. Our willingness to help others in some way becomes the proof that we have matured and grown as a result of our grief journey. No one can comfort a widow like another widow, just as no one can comfort someone who has lost a child like another parent who has lost a child.

Another "over the lips" activity is being or having a friend who will listen. A person can't share if no one is available to listen. A willing listener might just be the most important element. A friend who sticks close and is willing to be available at a moment's notice during extremely low times is invaluable. A friend that will listen, listen, and listen some more. Even if that person hears the same story over and over again, they are still willing to listen. Sometimes that friend doesn't have to say anything. They don't need any wise words in response. They just need to be willing to listen. Having someone to talk to when you are hurting is priceless. This helps the bereaved person "actualize the loss." As someone shares their grief story, they are able to process their grief and allow it to become a part of their new reality. They slowly accept or reconcile their grief into their present life and begin building a new life without the person who died. They don't forget the person they lost; they merely gain a new, mature perspective. They live their lives physically without the person who passed, but their memories of that person live on in their hearts and continue to enrich their lives.

Through the Fingertips

Another practical thing you can do in your work of mourning is write about how you feel. Some people are more comfortable writing about their feelings than talking about them. Writing is particularly important when you don't have someone to talk to. This written expression is also called journaling. It doesn't have to be anything formal, just a way to help transfer your feelings out of your head and heart and onto the page as a written expression of mourning. No one else needs to read it. Journaling is what you are feeling today, the sadness you are experiencing, and what triggered those feelings.

Date your journal entries, so you can measure your progress later. Journaling helps you look back and measure your grief journey by seeing how you have worked through your intense emotions. You can look back a week, a month, or a year and compare how you felt and dealt with an issue that day. This allows you to compare your present feelings to your past journal entries. You see your own maturation, growth, and healing as you processed pain through your grief journey over time. You can look back and be encouraged by your progress in your work of mourning. Many people have even turned their grief journals into books.

Some talented people express themselves through writing poetry. Music is also great if you are able to write music or play a musical instrument. Music can be very calming and can touch your heart.

Some old hymns are an expression of grief and how the Lord brought the songwriter through it. An example is the old hymn "It Is Well With My Soul," by Horatio Spafford. Spafford had a son who died of scarlet fever in 1870 and then lost much of his real estate holdings in the great Chicago fire of 1871. In 1873 he decided his family should take a vacation and go to England. At the last moment, due to pressing business concerns, he sent his family ahead of him on a steamship. The boat was struck by another vessel and sank, drowning his remaining four children, ages two to eleven. Only his wife survived. When he received his wife's telegram, "Saved alone," he set off at once to be reunited with her. During that voyage, he asked the captain to show him the very spot where the ship went down when they passed by. It is said that Spafford returned to his cabin and then wrote the hymn, "It Is Well With My Soul."

CHAPTER 21

——————⌖——————

Good Grief... Bad Grief

Not many of us could come to that level of faith to write a hymn that has lasted for generations, but with God all things are possible. God has a "big-picture view" that only He can see and understand. Only He knows what His purposes are for the future and the role we play in it. As we all experience our grief journeys, it is reassuring to know we can experience the Lord's unique comfort for each of us individually. Even though we moan and mourn our losses, wondering why they happen, God has a big-picture perspective that can become a positive reality only as we grow through our grief. We still will hurt, cry, and struggle along our grief journey, but we can still emerge as better, more mature people who are willing to help others.

Think of it in terms of a crucible or a hot furnace for precious metals. It's as if we are refined by the fire as we go through the furnace of grief, refined like precious metal, emerging as pure gold in the end. We emerge as better people for having gone through this process. Something positive can come out of a tragedy, although it may take some time to gain this perspective.

It's up to us whether we allow our grief to progress toward what I call "good grief." Good grief is not that we forget our grief but that our grief matures in a healthy manner to allow us to be used for what the Lord calls "good." It doesn't mean we won't cry and have moments of sadness. Such things are inevitable. It means, with the Lord's help, we can overcome grief's grip on us. We can receive the Lord's hand of comfort and pass it on to others.

The alternative to what I call "good grief" is "bad grief," which is nothing less than bondage. Grief can hold you hostage. Bad-grief-bondage is where the bereaved has made no effort to become seasoned, refined, or matured into a better person as a result of their grief journey. They have just given up and are unwilling to grow. Their grief has consumed them, and they have allowed it to do so. I compare it to being dropped into a deep lake (bereavement) where the choice is to sink or swim. Instead of doing the hard work of mourning (swimming), they choose to do nothing and stay in that place of "self-pity" and sink. This person chooses to live in the dark closet of grief, not allowing any light to shine in. Some people find this to be a safe place where they don't have to do any of the work of mourning. Like any work, mourning can be painful, difficult, and unpleasant. These people seem stuck in their grief and can't or won't see a future where they can mature and grow as people. They think their lives are over. They want everyone to feel sorry for them and their situation.

Their comfort is the sympathy they can muster up from others who will hear their complaints. Unfortunately, these people repel people around them rather than bless them. However, even if they make a small attempt to bless someone, it is at least a step in the right direction. This is another situation where you can choose your choices, but you can't choose the consequences of your choices. Many times you can help choose the path of your grief journey, good grief toward freedom or bad grief toward bondage. Are you willing to do the hard work of mourning to move in the direction of God's blessing?

Romans 8:37–39 (NLT)

No, despite all these things, overwhelming victory is ours through Christ, who loved us. And I am convinced that nothing can ever separate us from God's love. Neither death nor life, neither angels nor demons, neither our fears for today nor our worries about tomorrow—not even the powers of hell can separate us from God's love. No power in the sky above or in the earth below—indeed, nothing in all creation will ever be able to separate us from the love of God that is revealed in Christ Jesus our Lord.

Pondering Life and Service:

CHAPTER 22

———————⋉———————

Gaining the Proper Perspective

I t's not a matter of what we think; the important question is, what does God think? God's perspective is the only one that really matters. People dream up all kinds of far-fetched Ideas. Through the centuries, people continue to think they are the best and brightest and have all the answers, but today people have been deceived into thinking they can abandon biblical history and God's institution and announce they have reached the pinnacle of knowledge, morality, social structure, and political correctness.

God is the timeless Creator, and we must learn, study, and play by His rules of the game of life. Unfortunately, many people choose to believe a lie just because that's what the current culture teaches, believes, or thinks is the easiest answer to hear. Someone once said that if you tell a lie often enough, people will begin to believe it. Scripture teaches that Satan is the father of lies. Maybe that's why some lies seem so well-orchestrated and are quickly absorbed by the dark elements of our culture. Even some people who refer to themselves as churchgoers don't know what Scripture teaches on the subject of salvation and the entrance requirements to heaven.

When a hospice patient or a family member wanted to know what I thought or what the Bible had to say, I had the freedom to share openly with them. I helped them to understand the biblical teaching, that we all have gone astray at some point in our lives and need a Savior to save us.

Romans 3:23 (ESV)

...for all have sinned and fall short of the glory of God,

None of us are perfect. When my children and grandchildren were born, not one of them needed to be taught how to be selfish, angry, hateful, or fight their siblings. They all came with that sinful nature built in, as did all generations going back to Adam and Eve in the garden. A parent or grandparent's challenge is to give their best effort to train children up, teaching and modeling godly values and virtues as they grow. We all have seen what a modern culture of kids without a godly, biblical baseline of values and virtues looks like. They believe lies rather than the truth and have no moral compass for a stable life that has any traditional common sense. They quickly absorb and put into practice the lies that are taught to them. That's why Jesus came to earth in the form of a baby born from a virgin in a humble barn, the true story of Christmas we celebrate each year. Even though he was God in the flesh, Jesus grew up and experienced life as a human, just like us. It takes the Holy Spirit to fully grasp and understand the depth of all of this. The bottom line is that God loves us and wants us to connect with Him today and not wait until we think it's our time to die.

John 1:14 (NLT)

So the Word became human and made his home among us. He was full of unfailing love and faithfulness. And we have seen his glory, the glory of the Father's one and only Son.

Jesus became the humblest of humans to know what we experience and ultimately pay the price for our sin. Even though Jesus lived a sinless, perfect life and was innocent, he was willing to be punished as a criminal for us as part of His great plan to bridge the spiritual gap from unholy to holy. Even in His innocence, Jesus was willing to be executed in the worst-possible way (crucifixion) to be a substitute for the punishment for our sin, which we all deserve. This is the good news of the gospel: our debt of sin was paid by Christ, and His righteousness was credited to us. That great exchange of grace comes not by any work we do but by our step of faith in trusting in Jesus as our personal redeemer.

Ephesians 2:8–9 (NLT)

God saved you by his grace when you believed. And you can't take credit for this; it is a gift from God. Salvation is not a reward for the good things we have done, so none of us can boast about it.

We need to pause, study, and "chew" on this passage for a while. We must let it sink into our minds to fully grasp what was done for us and why the God of the universe was willing to do it.

Each of us must come to the place before God where He has our undivided, personal attention, and we realize our need for Him. Going to church on its own doesn't do it. We also can't ever do enough good things to work our way to heaven. How good is good enough to be considered a good person? Certainly, none of us are good looking enough, rich enough, educated enough, or have the proper family lineage to earn it. Then there's all the sin (past and present) in our lives that no one knows about but God. All of us need the grace and mercy of a savior to save us. We must honestly search our hearts before God.

We all were created with a place in our heart reserved for a one-on-one relationship with God, but many times we choose to fill that "God-shaped void" with something else. No family members can decide for us to follow Jesus, nor can anyone force us to believe. God loves us and gives us a free will to choose whether to love Him in return. Again, God doesn't want us to have religion but a personal, daily relationship with Him, a meaningful connection to Him in our lives that only comes by having that one-on-one, growing relationship with Jesus Christ .

I used to tell patients that going to church or church membership alone doesn't make you a Christian any more than walking into a garage makes you a Cadillac. God knows our hearts.

CHAPTER 23

————————⌖————————

Choosing to Believe Truth or a Lie

As a hospice chaplain, there are no do-overs when you're honored to be at the bedside of a dying patient as that person takes his or her last breath in this world. Just as the curtain comes down at the end of a performance, so does the curtain of life when death occurs. All the family connections, memories, and meaningful relationships come to an absolute end, whether we like it or not. Nothing more can be done to change any detail of our lives. What's done is done. Thus, as a hospice chaplain, I often prayed that I would be able to bless someone in a way that would make a meaningful difference, that God would use me to make an impact on them in their final days or hours.

After a patient's death, hospice chaplains—or anyone, for that matter—should reflect on the experience and ask themselves a series of questions, such as: Was all of this worthwhile? Could I have changed anything to make a more meaningful difference in this patient's life? Were my efforts good enough?

Of course, many of these thoughts and questions can't really be answered on this side of heaven. Whether you are a chaplain or not, the important thing to consider is that any reflection about your actions becomes an exercise to challenge you to grow and mature, to become a better person. Striving to be a better person is a conscious choice.

As we think about our lives and reflect upon our words, actions, and experiences, we must be willing to honestly explore our own life questions. It's easy to just continue to slide on, year after year, avoiding change. Doing nothing is easy, but then we wonder why life never changes positively for us.

As a grandfather now, my advice to those who are younger is that we all should stop to ponder these important questions about life. Maturity at any age happens according to the steps we take (or don't take) in response to our honest answers to these questions about life. Such questions should bring us to an important fork in the road where change can happen. We may not like what we see, and it may be too painful to deal with any of these answers on our own, but a self-examination of our motives and of who is really guiding our lives is the first step toward making important, positive changes in our lives. The changes I've made in response to such self-examination are reflected in this book.

I'm happy to report that as I look back at my life, it's clear to me that the Lord desires to help steer our lives. It took me a while to figure it all out, but I know that God wants to guide us in a direction that honors Him and truly blesses us beyond our wildest imagination. That's what part of this book is all about. But there is a secret to success along the way toward self-improvement and growth. That secret is revealed when we surrender our lives to the one who knows every hair on our heads. Surrendering control of our lives is a foreign concept to us. We spend most of our lives wanting to be the boss, the captain of our own ship. We have had parents, teachers, bosses, and the government all telling us what to do. Now we want to run our lives our own way and live to the fullest. At least that's what we think or hope for.

But this concept of surrendering to the Lord doesn't really go against our desire to live life to the fullest. The Lord desires the best for us as well. The surrender part comes in when we acknowledge that He is God, and we are not. God has our best interests at heart. We must acknowledge that God is our Creator and that He created each of us for a specific purpose. When we learn to pursue this God-ordained purpose, we truly find the fullest life possible. We start looking at our lives from God's perspective rather than our own.

The grandfatherly wisdom I want to pass along is that becoming a better person only happens as a result of intent—when we choose to let God work in us. It becomes a question of whether to serve yourself or to open your mind and heart to let God lovingly mold you into who He wants you to be. It's a choice to walk with God or continue to walk on your own. God allows us this choice. Serving ourselves is easy and comes naturally. We all want what we want and selfishly go for it all, getting upset when things don't go our way.

This exciting new thought process begins when we learn to think beyond ourselves and into the lives of others. As I look back at my life, I realize a reflective question that you might want to ask yourself today is this: are you trying to make a difference in someone else's life? Allow me to elaborate on this for a moment as you think about your interactions in life.

Some of the greatest blessings and rewards in life come from actions or careers where someone is purposely trying to make a positive impact in someone else's life. Even just a touch of kindness or hope, no matter how small, done for someone else helps to change lives in ways we often don't realize. Having this mindset can result in a significant difference every day.

I have often thought this challenge would make a difference not only in my life but in our entire nation. If everyone made some effort, even a little attempt to be kind and loving, the world would be a better, less selfish place. We would see a definite cause and effect as this positive hope and encouragement was passed on.

I know it's easy to pursue a career believing the reward is all about making a large income with all the toys that go along with it, especially when you are living as if God doesn't exist. This demonstrates our natural tendency to be totally self-absorbed, selfishly thinking that it's all about us and what we want in life, even being willing to steal or step on others to get it. Working for a living is important, and earning a good income is certainly something God wants us to do. However, doing so becomes a problem when other people's lives aren't considered and where money and selfishness become the center of our lives. We totally miss a blessing far greater than any physical or monetary reward that's available to us.

As a hospice chaplain, I have never seen anyone take any of life's toys with them to their deathbeds thinking they would get to keep them when they died. This seems to be the deceptive American dream that money, toys, and power are the main rewards of life. Many people chasing this dream quickly find their lives spent and never realize they missed some of the most important blessings in life. I've seen many people come to the end of their life before they examine their hearts. Some never do.

It's all too common for people to live with this selfish mentality of thinking God should have no part in it, foolishly believing God doesn't exist because they don't see Him or think He does. They rebel against anyone who knows the truth about God and tries to share this good news with them. They think shutting God and His followers out of their lives can separate God from His own creation. Unfortunately, our culture tries to support this. People have believed a lie, and no one has taught them what actual truth is. Lies have been repeated for so long by so many people that people now accept lies as the basis for their truth. They don't know any different. Jesus taught that Satan is the father of lies and that God's truth needs to be discovered.

John 8:44–45 (NLT)

For you are the children of your father the devil, and you love to do the evil things he does. He was a murderer from the beginning. He has always hated the truth, because there is no truth in him. When he lies, it is consistent with his character; for he is a liar and the father of lies. So when I tell the truth, you just naturally don't believe me.

Some see the world being on autopilot with Mother Nature being in control and humankind as the ultimate climate maker. Or they selfishly desire to be the most powerful one in their world. Just because lies are convenient or easy to believe certainly doesn't nullify God's truth. Not believing in God's sovereignty is like saying, "I didn't vote for the president, I don't know or like the president, and I haven't actually seen the president; therefore, the president doesn't exist."

Pondering the important questions of life should be done today as opposed to waiting to reflect on your deathbed. Waiting until then to ponder the "would've, could've, and should've" decisions lead to a truly wasted life. Don't contemplate who God is; discover who God is by exploring what the Bible says about Him. There's a reason why for centuries so many people have proclaimed the Bible as God's Word, as evidenced by their changed lives. Further evidence is the opposition to the Bible over the centuries. If it were just a plain, powerless book, why has it transformed millions of lives for good—mine being one of them—and lasted for centuries? There must be a reason why the enemy of our souls wants the Holy Bible banned, burned, and unread. Truth must be examined and never hidden.

Have you've spent the time you've been given wisely? Will the time investments of your life translate into a "dividend" that is meaningful or worthwhile? Has your life made a real difference to someone else? Can you look back and see God's fingerprints on your life? Have you been able to discover God's love for you by His definitions of forgiveness, judgement, and salvation? As much as we would like to make up our own rules for the game of life, we must come to the end of ourselves and realize that only God's rules really count. Certainly, these are heavy thoughts to consider, but they are worth pondering—if you dare.

CHAPTER 24

—————◇×————

Loving Foundation for Serving

I n my career as a hospice chaplain, the Lord taught me that making an effort to make a difference in someone else's life blessed my own life beyond measure. It gave my life purpose and meaning, I would have never had it any other way I think this principle can be applied to many jobs in life. Being a blessing to someone else blesses you in return. What a wonderful world we would have if everyone strived to be a blessing to others. Even the smallest blessing is a dose of love and hope into others' lives, but that love must start somewhere. If we are honest, it doesn't start with us. We all tend to be selfish and want what we want. We want the blessing, but we often aren't willing to be the blessing.

Real love starts with God, and our willingness to accept His love for ourselves is the true beginning of change. When we feel God's touch in our lives, we willingly pass God's love on to those we interact with. We become a true reflection of God's love to others.

Once we know the Lord, we learn that we can't serve and honor Him unless we have the goal of loving others in some manner. It's not something we have to do; we want to do it because it brings us joy. Jesus made it noticeably clear that living a self-absorbed life is not a blessing to Him or anyone else. Blessing and serving God means learning how to devote ourselves to loving God and loving one another. It requires pre-meditation on our part. Jesus made it clear that this isn't the Lord's suggestion but a commandment. Jesus demonstrated His intentional love for us. It's to be the foundation for us to be able to serve others. Love from the heart is the key to making any positive change in ourselves and society as a whole. Love can't be legislated, nor can anyone be bullied into doing it. Love is a heart issue. As we walk closely with Jesus, it becomes a natural consequence to loving the Lord with all our heart, soul, and mind.

Matthew 22:37–40 (NLT)

Jesus replied, "'You must love the LORD your God with all your heart, all your soul, and all your mind.' This is the first and greatest commandment. A second is equally important: 'Love your neighbor as yourself.' The entire law and all the demands of the prophets are based on these two commandments."

If we are obedient to His command to love, Jesus uses us to pass His love on to others in this hurting world. As we strive to love God with our heart, soul, and mind, He uses us as His hands and feet in the small part of the world we live in each day. Each of us has our own unique world where the Lord has placed us to serve Him in some manner. He created each of us (uniquely) to serve Him. He uses our talents, abilities, education, and even our past hurtful history to prepare us to help others. Even if a person is hurting today, God has created, equipped, and prepared that person to bless someone in the future as a result of that damaging experience. God can turn around anything Satan intends to harm us with and use it to demonstrate His love through us. No one can help someone who is going through a tough experience like someone who has been through it themselves. They can testify to God's love, healing power, and provision based on their own firsthand experience.

Not everyone is a chaplain, but we all can come alongside someone who is hurting as if we were a chaplain. It's just a matter of our willingness to care about someone else in some fashion. The Lord brings neighbors, coworkers, family members, and friends into our lives and wants us to learn to lean on Him, so we can love and help others. To be blessed ourselves, we need to be a blessing to others. Our willingness to do so is the first step in this effort. It's learning to have a servant-like heart, a heart that is committed to the truth of loving the Lord and trusting Him for the strength and power we don't have. Knowing we don't have what it takes is paramount in this growth process. In any unique and difficult situation, our goal is to allow God to work through us to accomplish what only He can do. God is already busy working in someone else's life in some way. We just need to have the willingness and mindset to join God in His work and what He wants to accomplish through us to help someone else. It's not a matter of thinking God should join us in what we think should happen.

CHAPTER 25

———————⚮———————

This Isn't All There Is

John 3:16–17 (NLT)

For God loved the world so much that he gave his one and only Son, so that everyone who believes in him will not perish but have eternal life. God sent his Son into the world not to judge the world, but to save the world through him.

W hen I had the opportunity, I also reminded people that this life is not all there is. Preparing for death is preparing for eternal life. When we think about it, none of us knows when our last day or breath will be. Each of us must live in a state of readiness to meet our maker at any time. Accidents happen every day, but God has a plan for our lives from birth to our dying breath.

Psalm 139:15–16 (NLT)

You watched me as I was being formed in utter seclusion, as I was woven together in the dark of the womb. You saw me before I was born. Every day of my life was recorded in your book. Every moment was laid out before a single day had passed.

For those who have reconciled their hearts to Jesus, there is all of eternity, a place called heaven that we can all look forward to. It's a place where the wrongs of this world are made right. Heaven is where we will see our loved ones who knew Jesus, a place where there are no more tears, pain, or suffering.

Revelation 7:17 (NLT)

For the Lamb on the throne will be their Shepherd. He will lead them to springs of life-giving water. And God will wipe every tear from their eyes."

Heaven is also a place where we could be going with a commanding shout, with the voice of the archangel, and with the trumpet call of God. Getting there requires a willingness to let God be God and not think He has to operate according to our timeline.

1 Thessalonians 4:13–18 (NLT)

And now, dear brothers and sisters, we want you to know what will happen to the believers who have died so you will not grieve like people who have no hope. For since we believe that Jesus died and was raised to life again, we also believe that when Jesus returns, God will bring back with him the believers who have died. We tell you this directly from the Lord: We who are still living when the Lord returns will not meet him ahead of those who have died. For the Lord himself will come down from heaven with a commanding shout, with the voice of the archangel, and with the trumpet call of God. First, the Christians who have died will rise from their graves. Then, together with them, we who are still alive and remain on the earth will be caught up in the clouds to meet the Lord in the air. Then we will be with the Lord forever. So encourage each other with these words.

Knowing who Paid the Price for Admission

The world's wishful thinking that everyone is going to heaven is not what the Bible teaches. Chaplains need to have a firm grasp of this reality. According to Scripture, heaven is a place where the admission price was paid by Jesus, not by us or anyone else. We can't just analyze our thoughts regarding heaven according to our own "warm and fuzzy" human emotions. It goes much deeper than that. There's no solid biblical basis for the belief that everyone goes to heaven without any entrance requirements because we think that's what a loving God would do.

The good news is, God has provided the greatest way to heaven, and admission is free. However, we still must play by God's rules for admission because He is the holy God of the universe. There's a big divide between this holy, righteous, all-knowing God and unrighteous, sinful humankind. We need a spiritual bridge to take us from our sinfulness across to our holy God. Because of God's great love for us, Jesus himself is that spiritual bridge to help us cross the gap we can't cross on our own.

This means that only by personally acknowledging that Jesus died for us and paid the ultimate price for us can any of us obtain our free ticket to heaven. Each person needs to seriously ponder this provision of God's grace and mercy for all of us and not just dismiss it all as a part of theology or religion. Anything less misses the significance of the personal sacrifice of Jesus Christ and the shedding of His blood for us on the cross as His ultimate gift of love.

It's a choice that must be deeply evaluated by everyone. Making no decision or deciding to follow something other than Jesus is the wrong choice. According to Scripture, this becomes a default decision to forfeit heaven.

Romans 1:20 (NLT)

For ever since the world was created, people have seen the earth and sky. Through everything God made, they can clearly see his invisible qualities—his eternal power and divine nature. So they have no excuse for not knowing God.

The Lord desires us to choose to follow Him daily, to live life to its fullest today and not just as a preparation for dying. Nor does He want us to quickly say the words of salvation just to claim our "fire insurance." He knows our hearts. The Lord wants us to live a lifestyle of faith that's more than being called "religious" by those who watch our lives and give us that label. God doesn't want us to just have religion; God wants us to have a relationship with Him that's not necessarily tied to any particular denomination. There's a huge difference that casual observers of life and faith often miss, including many so-called Christians.

We all must come to a point of personal surrender and realize that God is God, and we are not. Our perspective on our relationship with God is important to our personal connection with Him because it shapes our hearts and minds' development of this relationship. We shouldn't think of our relationship with God as a "giant-ant," "master-slave," or "boss-employee" kind of relationship. God desires a loving father-child relationship where the heavenly parent already knows what His children need before being asked. He wants His children to grow into an intimate relationship with Him as we seek and ask Him for the help we need in our lives, help that only He can truly give us.

Developing a close relationship with God involves a healthy fear of knowing He alone is God and orders life, and He isn't a heavenly Santa who does whatever we ask. It also involves the realization that He loves us individually and uniquely, and he gives His gifts to us through Jesus, gifts that we can't ever earn or buy. Being a Christians means being part of a loving relationship where we do our part to nurture our relationship with Him through reading His Word (the Bible) and praying with an openness of our hearts. Someone once described it this way: Man says, "Show me and I'll believe." God says, "Believe me, and I'll show you." Having a relationship with God means having a connection to Him where He is able to shape our perspective on life, guide our priorities, and show us the steps that he wants us to take. We sense His loving connection through His Spirit and learn to hear Him speak to our hearts. He wants to glorify Himself through our lives as we learn to trust Him in a mature, healthy relationship with Him.

1 Peter 5:5–7 (NLT)

"God opposes the proud but favors the humble." So humble yourselves under the mighty power of God, and at the right time he will lift you up in honor. Give all your worries and cares to God, for he cares about you.

CHAPTER 26

———————✂———————

Limited Opportunities to Make a Choice

B eing in an occupation that deals with death, you ponder the seriousness of life from both a human perspective as well as what God's perspective must be. Of course, God's perspective is only known if we read and study the bible as a part of our daily lives. Through faith, we learn how important God's grace and mercy are to our lives and we can't take it casually. When we come to the end of life, either our name is written in the Lamb's book of life or it's not. There's no third choice that I can see in scripture.

Revelation 21:27 (NLT)

Nothing evil will be allowed to enter, nor anyone who practices shameful idolatry and dishonesty—but only those whose names are written in the Lamb's Book of Life.

The seriousness is that you can choose God's heaven or reject it; it's up to you. God allows you to be in charge of your ultimate destiny, but sometimes there is no second opportunity in life to reconsider or change your mind. There is a price to be paid for procrastinating in your relationship with God. The decision becomes as simple as choosing whether to be on the winning team or the losing team. Someone once said, "You can choose your choices, but you can't choose the consequences that come with each choice." It's like you choose which stack of dominoes will fall behind the choice you make of accepting Christ or rejecting Him.

Scripture states that the Holy Spirit must draw you, and you must respond. You can respond in only one of two ways.

1) Accept Jesus at his word. Acknowledge that He died for you, ask Him to forgive your sins, repent of your sins, and believe in faith, trusting Jesus Christ as your Savior.
2) Reject Jesus, His message, and His gift of salvation. With this decision, or with no decision at all, you forfeit God's grace and mercy of spending eternity in heaven with Him and all those who have believed the message of Jesus.

1 John 1:8–10 (NLT)

If we claim we have no sin, we are only fooling ourselves and not living in the truth.
But if we confess our sins to him, he is faithful and just to forgive us our sins and to cleanse us from all wickedness.
If we claim we have not sinned, we are calling God a liar and showing that his word has no place in our hearts.

Only Jesus can bring a hospice patient or anyone to the place of having hope despite having a terminal illness. If we honestly think about it, we all are terminal. We just don't know when our lives will end. Even though the current culture views such thinking as unnecessary or incredibly old fashioned, God says differently, and His truth is timeless. The ultimate question and challenge for all of us is this: which path will we follow? If today was your last day, what would your choice be? Is it door number one or number two?

Hebrews 13:8–9 (NLT)

Jesus Christ is the same yesterday, today, and forever. So do not be attracted by strange, new ideas. Your strength comes from God's grace, not from rules about food, which don't help those who follow them.

John 14:1–6 (NLT)

"Don't let your hearts be troubled. Trust in God, and trust also in me.
There is more than enough room in my Father's home. If this were not so, would I have told you that I am going to prepare a place for you?
When everything is ready, I will come and get you, so that you will always be with me where I am.
And you know the way to where I am going."
"No, we don't know, Lord," Thomas said. "We have no idea where you are going, so how can we know the way?"
Jesus told him, "I am the way, the truth, and the life. No one can come to the Father except through me.

Considerations for Being a Hospice Chaplain:

CHAPTER 27

———————⋈———————

How Do You Do What You Do?

Psalm 116:15 (ESV)

Precious in the sight of the LORD is the death of his saints.

As a hospice chaplain, I was often asked, "How can you do what you do? How can you deal with death and dying every day? Isn't it too depressing?"

The death of a follower of Jesus is precious to God. The circumstances and individuals involved in this personal experience play an important part in God's mission. Anyone considering becoming a hospice chaplain should share in a willingness to join God in the work He is already doing in the lives of dying Christians and their families.

The primary emotional consideration for a potential hospice chaplain is whether this is going to be just a job or if it's going to be a calling or a ministry. If it's just a job that you think you can do, you won't last long or be very effective. Overwhelming emotional questions and situations happen

131

frequently as you try to provide support to terminally ill individuals and their family members. These situations and questions are way bigger than you are, and you have no control over any of them, so there's no way you can handle them on your own.

In this occupation, you will face struggles and questions, such as: where does your strength come from to help others? How do you deal with all the emotional stress? How can you project calm into an emotionally difficult situation? How can you answer someone who is terminally ill and searching for truth and hope before they die? These questions can only be answered when there is a solid basis of truth from which to draw from. It isn't a matter of trying to be all things to all people. Without an openness and connection to God, you will develop a hardened heart just so you can do the job.

The Basis for Truth for Everyone: Fact or Fiction

Everyone thinks they have a form of truth in their life, even if it's based on a lie. Do you really know if your life is based on fact or fiction? It's through self-examination and an evaluation of our definition of truth that we discover whether our lives are truly based on the rock-solid foundation of God's perspective. A meaningful life needs to be set on a firm foundation of truth that can weather the storms of life. Not doing so is like a carpenter who refuses to use a plumbline or a square edge to build a house and then wonders why the finished house is not square with nothing fitting right. Scripture explains it as "everyone doing what is right in their own eyes."

Proverbs 21:2 (NLT)

People may be right in their own eyes, but the LORD examines their heart.

What is the foundation or baseline for truth? It comes down to discovering that only God, as the Creator of the universe, is the absolute source for truth. God's truth is not relative to anything else. Your present truth could be the basis of what you think, as informed by your feelings, your education, or what the current culture teaches. You might desire to be current, to go along with current political correctness or the trendy thinking of the day. Every other source of so-called truth seems to change quickly like the latest fashion or political movement. It's daring to allow the Lord to examine your heart and to study His word to determine what is (or what should be) your source of your truth.

1 Peter 1:24–25 (NLT)

As the Scriptures say, "People are like grass; their beauty is like a flower in the field. The grass withers and the flower fades. But the word of the Lord remains forever." And that word is the Good News that was preached to you.

All of this needs to be evaluated against what God defines as timeless truth through His Holy Bible. This goes against all human logic, and it requires courage to seek and explore beyond the prevalent thought of the day. It's certainly important for anyone who wants to live an authentic, meaningful, blessed life.

An effective hospice chaplain or pastor senses if the Lord is directing his or her path. If you have a daily walk with the Lord, He will give you the leading, inclination, or sense of direction to serve Him as you serve others. As we step out in faith to serve the Lord, the Lord begins to direct our path, often through other godly individuals and encouragement. Someone once described it this way to me: "It's easier to steer a car that's moving than one that is standing still."

It's important to believe that God has prepared (and is preparing) you for your mission for God's glory, not your own. Look for a confirmation or affirmation in your spirit that your mission or your direction is the one that God has planned for you. As you step out in service to the Lord, He will direct your path, opening and closing doors along the way.

You must operate on the Lord's truth and strength, so you can confidently pass along or reflect God's truth and strength to those who are looking to you for it. It's the only way to find joy despite all the adversities of life. It's also important to know how to access truth and strength, which you don't have on your own.

CHAPTER 28

———⤬———

Victory Over Death?

Like it or not, death is part of life. Your personal reflection of death and its place in our world is important to being able to understand how God has placed death as a major part of the cycle of life. From a human perspective, death is the most dreaded thing for everyone. The question that needs to be answered for anyone is, do you believe there is victory over death? If so, who achieved that victory? How does that victory affect you as well as hospice patients?

Hebrews 2:14–15 (NLT)

Because God's children are human beings—made of flesh and blood—the Son also became flesh and blood. For only as a human being could he die, and only by dying could he break the power of the devil, who had the power of death. Only in this way could he set free all who have lived their lives as slaves to the fear of dying.

1 Corinthians 15:55–57 (NLT)

"O death, where is your victory? O death, where is your sting?" For sin is the sting that results in death, and the law gives sin its power. But thank God. He gives us victory over sin and death through our Lord Jesus Christ.

Early in my role as a chaplain, I realized that on my own power and ability, I quickly came up short and was overwhelmed in dealing with death and dying. Even though I felt I had a heart for it, even a calling, I needed more. I needed God's strength and perspective. But how?

Walking the hospice-death journey is a heavy, difficult, and emotionally draining experience for anyone. It also brings up unresolved grief from your past that must continually be processed. Grief pain can accumulate as we try to stuff it down rather than deal with it. Grief must be worked through at the heart and head levels.

As you deal with others' pain and grief, your own grief pain will surface quite often. As a chaplain, I was forced to deal with my own pain and grief constantly. Some chapters in this book describe that pain. A chaplain's grief pain compounds and is mixed in with the current grief pain from losing hospice patients that he or she grows to love. It's all part of having a sensitive heart and caring about others. It's not a bad thing, but you must be aware of grief that can accumulate, leaving you vulnerable and overwhelmed. It also could cause you to harden your heart as a defense against grief.

Chaplains miss their hospice patients and even mourn them when they die. That's a good thing because it means you don't have a hardened heart and that you really do care. I used to have a large clear glass container in the office that

I used as a personal memorial for our office. I placed a colored glass stone into the container each time a patient died. The jar represented all the hospice patients we had served. Over time when I saw the large jar full of those colored glass stones, it represented the accumulation of all the meaningful efforts achieved by many hospice workers. Each of those hospice workers, working together as a team, made a significant difference in the end-of-life care for each of those patients and their families. A full jar was symbolic of making a difference in the lives of others. Such a healthy, positive perspective is important.

To be effective and have the necessary strength to help others, I needed to experience the Lord's healing and stability in my own life. To come alongside and support someone else, I needed to know how to support them, which meant tapping into the power of Christ, so I could be a conduit of that power to them. I needed Christ to set me free and work through me as well as those I was trying to help. I could not be a slave to the fear of dying and grief. Otherwise, I would pass this fear on to my patients.

CHAPTER 29

———————⟡———————

Hang onto the Vine

In a continuing effort to answer the question, "How do you do what you do?", I'd like to share a simple illustration that Jesus gives in the Bible that became profound, meaningful, and so important to me in trying to be an effective chaplain. It removed the pressure of carrying others' burdens and trying to operate my ministry on the limited emotional "fuel" in my tank. It took the weight off my shoulders and placed it where it needed to be, on the Lord's shoulders. It became more of a relational lesson than an intellectual one, a matter of knowing the difference between walking with the Lord and " just knowing about the Lord. The lesson is found in John 15. This profound lesson is so simple but so hard at the same time. I think that's why Jesus gave us this simple graphic illustration to help us grasp its deep meaning and ultimate benefit for our lives. It's an illustration that I needed to have that connection to Jesus by "hanging onto the vine" (Jesus), the true source of power. This simple picture was like a light bulb turning on in my mind. This visualization of the vine and the branches can be applied to anyone who desires to tap into God's strength with the end result of bearing God-given fruit and making a difference in someone else's life.

John 15:1–10 (NLT)

I am the true grapevine, and my Father is the gardener. He cuts off every branch of mine that doesn't produce fruit, and he prunes the branches that do bear fruit so they will produce even more. You have already been pruned and purified by the message I have given you. Remain in me, and I will remain in you. For a branch cannot produce fruit If it is severed from the vine, and you cannot be fruitful unless you remain in me. Yes, I am the vine; you are the branches. Those who remain in me, and I in them, will produce much fruit. For apart from me you can do nothing. Anyone who does not remain in me is thrown away like a useless branch and withers. Such branches are gathered into a pile to be burned. But if you remain in me and my words remain in you, you may ask for anything you want, and it will be granted. When you produce much fruit, you are my true disciples. This brings great glory to my Father. I have loved you even as the Father has loved me. Remain in my love. When you obey my commandments, you remain in my love, just as I obey my Father's commandments and remain in his love.

Being fruitful wasn't under my power. Jesus' story about grapes only coming from the grapevine was a personal revelation and a great relief. It wasn't supposed to be under my power, even when I foolishly thought it should be. Only God could produce the fruit he wants to produce in others' lives.

Only He can accomplish what he wants to accomplish. I just need to be flexible and to be His useful conduit for his fruit-bearing energy to flow. Jesus is the grapevine (the true source of energy), and my connection to Him is the key. I just need to remind myself to stay connected to the grapevine (Jesus). Actually, the most important piece of this illustration to remember is the last part of verse 5. Realizing that apart from Jesus, *I can do nothing.* No connection to the vine, no fruit.

In my work with hospice, there was only one way I could come to grips with uncontrollable people and circumstances. I needed to be willing to be flexible and available to the one (God) who does control circumstances and convict hearts. If I was going to help bear any fruit as a chaplain, I needed to remain connected to the true source of truth, wisdom, and power. A connection to Jesus through the Holy Spirit, allowing Him to work through me to accomplish what He wants to accomplish is paramount for success. It becomes a personal application of yielding to Him and leaving the door open for His strength to be visible. It's giving God room to accomplish what He wants to do through us. Bearing fruit, staying connected to the vine, gives God glory.

Where the Rubber Meets the Road

As a hospice chaplain, this was a true test of my faith, trusting Him to do the work was where the rubber met the road in my ministry. This private test of a working faith was exercised as I worked with many people over time. An example of this working faith was sometimes simply learning to keep my mouth shut and giving the Lord time to work in someone's heart. I might say something to plant a seed in someone's mind, but only the Holy Spirit can make it sprout and take root. Sometimes it was asking a question and being quiet long enough for someone to think about it and start talking first. Letting silence happen isn't always easy. Sometimes we think we need to talk all the time to fill the space. However, silence gives the Holy Spirit time to penetrate hearts and minds. In counseling, it's hard to let silence happen, but it's particularly important in the Holy Spirit's work. The Holy Spirit's work is what is needed for people to share their hearts and take conversations where they need to go. Many times it is like priming an old pump. Once you get it started, meaningful discussion will flow. When the chaplain admits he or she is weak, God is glorified to show Himself strong. I learned to acknowledge my weakness and my need for His strength.

2 Corinthians 12:9–10 (NLT)

Each time he said, "My grace is all you need. My power works best in weakness." So now I am glad to boast about my weaknesses, so that the power of Christ can work through me. That's why I take pleasure in my weaknesses, and in the insults, hardships, persecutions, and troubles that I suffer for Christ. For when I am weak, then I am strong.

CHAPTER 30

———⋈———

Walking into a Buzzsaw

Without God, I could do nothing. In many patient and family homes, I knew I was walking into an emotional "buzzsaw." Emotions would be running high with grief or anger. At times I didn't know what I could say or do to help. I was fearful of making things worse. Many times I went into a home where people didn't know me, and I didn't know them. Sometimes I would be asked to go into a home to help "fix" or "manage" an emotionally difficult situation. I needed to be the one who could bring calm into such emotional situations. I needed to help families work through their initial grief and reach the point where I could allow the funeral home to come and remove the body. This took time, patience, and wisdom, all of which I needed God to provide.

At such times I needed to prepare myself emotionally as I drove to a patient's home. These situations were way bigger than I was able to control. My own efforts were not good enough. In preparation, I would literally raise my hand and pray as if I were hanging on to the vine (John 15:5) and ask God to work through me, to give me the words and scriptures

I needed to be fruitful and make a difference as only God could. I was often amazed at what came out of my mouth that truly helped someone. There were moments where God had me at the right time and right place to demonstrate His amazing, providential work. He was well aware of the situation and was in total control. Many times it became overwhelmingly evident to me that the Holy Spirit had indeed "showed up and showed off." Some of these God-glorifying stories are in this book. It wasn't a matter of asking God to join me in my work but making sure I was joining God is what He was already doing in the lives of others.

God often brought scriptures to my mind during conversations, or the Holy Spirit revealed a matter in a counseling situation to help guide the discussion. His Spirit would give me discernment to see the root issue in someone's life, a major issue that needed to be addressed or prayed about. Then we would ask the Lord to speak truth into that person's heart and their situation.

I was grateful that I learned it wasn't about me. It wasn't what great things I could do or say or needed to know. It was always about joining God in His work, in what He was already doing or preparing to do in someone else's life. It was God using me (allowing me) to be the answer to someone's prayer. It was the Lord allowing a hospice patient to have a last opportunity to get their heart right with God before they died. It was being a support system to caregivers or family members to encourage them at a difficult time, realizing it was all in His timing, power, and strength and not mine. Many times it seemed I was just along for the journey that God was already working out in someone else's life and death.

CHAPTER 31

———————⟨✕⟩———————

Bugs and Snakes

In an effort toward full disclosure, I want to pass along a not-so-obvious requirement to become a hospice chaplain: the ability to deal with a large amount of medical charting or documentation that has become a major part of our medical world today. Writing such documentation requires a great deal of time and energy. For me, this charting started in the early days as paper notes that I wrote by hand and then progressed over time to using portable laptops, then electronic tablets with a Bluetooth keyboard to type notes that were uploaded and synchronized to the company's main database.

When writing such documentation, chaplains need to paint a picture that provides their view of the hospice patient's terminal illness. Chaplains shouldn't include any personal notes regarding what patients tell them. It's merely a matter of observing the decline in the patient's illness and its effect on the patient and his or her family. The notes should also include the chaplain's supportive presence to the patient and family and any active-listening skills used to help everyone involved. The notes should also include evidence that supports these observations (pain, crying, anger, sadness, etc.). Such careful observation and note taking becomes an important skill in itself.

Nurses, physicians, and Medicare officials or surveyors often look at the chaplain's notes months later to evaluate, from the chaplain's perspective, a patient's eligibility to receive Medicare hospice benefit for payment of services. A hospice chaplain's documentation, along with all the hospice team notes, have been determining factors in this decision of whether Medicare funds were appropriately paid to a hospice organization. I often joked that being a hospice chaplain was like being a missionary in the jungle, and the documentation and paperwork were the "bugs and snakes" in the jungle that I had to tolerate to do my job.

Concluding Thoughts:

CHAPTER 32

———————✧———————

Honored to Meet Wonderful People

It was an honor to meet hundreds of people over the years whom I never would have met any other way. What a blessing to get to know these wonderful people at the end of their lives. I got to hear their stories, experiences, and personal memories, memories that would have disappeared when they died if not shared with me. I was privileged and honored that the Lord worked through me in my effort to make a positive difference in their lives. They definitely made a difference in my life that I will always cherish.

I was also blessed to know some of the most wonderful families and witness their selfless love and dedication in taking on the challenge of caring for their loved ones to the end. I saw children, grandchildren, nephews, and nieces honoring their fathers, mothers, grandmothers, grandfathers, uncles, and aunts by providing devoted care. Many times family members put their own lives on hold to provide necessary and sometimes unpleasant care and support. Some cleared out their living rooms to put up hospital beds for their loved ones. Others visited as often as they could when patients needed to go to a nursing home. I witnessed husbands and wives keeping their marriage vows of "until death do us part" even when dementia robbed the patient of any meaningful memories.

When I Die...

Over the years I have been with many hospice patients as they died, more patients than I can count. I have been honored to perform many funerals for patients and have served hundreds, maybe even thousands, of hospice patients. I often think of what it will be like when I die. I wonder if I might be greeted by a heavenly welcoming committee comprised of all the hospice patients I have served over the years who knew Jesus. Since I helped to see them off as they left this world for heaven, maybe they will all be there to greet me when it's my time to arrive. It's an emotional, overwhelming blessing to think of those hundreds of souls being there to greet me, along with the Lord Himself. It will truly take an eternity to talk to them all again.

I Have Worked with a Wonderful Staff

Over the years I had the privilege of working with wonderful aides, nurses, social workers, office staff, volunteers, and physicians. They were dedicated to helping patients and their families through the most difficult time of their lives. In the hospice offices where I worked, every morning we would have an update meeting (we called them "stand-up" meetings because they were supposed to be short) to discuss what had happened the day and night before in preparation for our current day's visits to patients. At the end of those meetings, I would take prayer requests and then pray for the staff for that day. I always felt led to pray that the Lord would use each of us to make a difference in the lives of the patients and their family members we would see, serve, and experience that day. In hospice, each day was filled with adventure, triumph, or tragedy as we all tried to do our jobs and make a difference despite difficult and often unpleasant circumstances.

CHAPTER 33

———◇———

The Last Day

My last day as a hospice chaplain came without me knowing it would be my last day. It was March 12, 2020. The world was starting to panic about all the rumors of COVID-19. The nursing home that I visited at least twice a week had started to quarantine certain sections of the building due to the flu. Within days it was discovered to have a major COVID outbreak. I felt I had been dodging the flu for a month due to several of our hospice patients and their family members coming down with it. I had been busy doing funerals and keeping an active schedule, visiting hospice patients and trying to keep myself as healthy as possible, including proper nutrition, rest, and washing and sanitizing my hands frequently between patients.

On March 12, 2020, I had a funeral to perform for a dear lady whom I had been seeing for over a year while also providing support to her daughter. The burial was going to be in a country cemetery, so I planned to see a hospice patient who lived within a mile of that cemetery following the graveside committal service.

On the morning of March 12, 2020, I was up at 6:00 a.m., as usual, to prepare for the busy day but was starting to feel unwell. "Lord, I can't make it through the day without your help and strength," I prayed.

I was at the office by 7:30, but following our stand-up meeting, I knew I was not going to make it without lying down. I told the RN supervisor I was going home to sleep for a couple of hours before I needed to be at the funeral home to do the service.

After my nap, I got up and put on my black suit to go do the funeral. Once again I prayed, "Lord, I'm weak, and I need your strength to finish the day." If you have ever heard the expression "fake it to make it" that was all I could do to make it through the funeral service as I trusted the Lord for strength.

At the cemetery, following the patient's burial, I thought, *Thank you, Jesus, I've made it this far.*

As mentioned, following the funeral, I had promised to see a patient who wasn't doing well and to provide support to his wife. I realized I may not have the opportunity again. The declining patient, despite having dementia, always responded well to my visits and prayers with him. His wife was always appreciative of my visits and support as well. I decided to visit them but to keep my distance and not make physical contact with them. Once again, I trusted the Lord to "fake it to make it."

The patient responded well to my visit, during which I was careful not to touch him or his wife, telling them I didn't want to spread any germs. As I left the house, all I could say was "Thank you, Jesus" because of what I was able to do that day.

I went straight home and went to bed, where I stayed for the next several days, unable to go to work. I don't think I have ever been that sick before. The national COVID shutdown was beginning to happen, so I just took vacation time and stayed home.

Everyone in the office, including me, was convinced I had COVID-19 because I was so sick. My wife was getting sick as well. I wouldn't have been surprised if I died, but I trusted the Lord, knowing the best was yet to come for me too.

A nurse friend in the hospital who found out how sick I had been called me and insisted that I be one of the first folks tested for the coronavirus at the hospital in Morgantown. My wife and I were tested, and thankfully, it was determined we both just had a bad case of the flu and not COVID-19. However, it took a full month before I had any strength again.

I had often said that I thought I would never retire and would be a chaplain for as long as I could. But we do have aging bodies and minds, and I certainly felt my own physical decline. But now I prayed, "Lord, do you want me to retire? May I retire?" I felt peaceful about it and decided to go ahead and retire on my sixty-sixth birthday. I never saw another hospice patient as a chaplain. As I reflected upon my career, I thought about the apostle Paul in his charge to Timothy when he said, "*I have fought the good fight, I have finished the race, and I have remained faithful*" (2 Timothy 4:7).

I am grateful for the ministry the Lord had shaped and prepared me for in that season of my life. I am grateful that He was able to use me and work through me in my efforts to make a difference in the lives of many hospice patients and their family members. The patients and families that I met and visited truly blessed and enriched my life. Now as I enter a new season, I once again claim John 15:5 and "hang onto the vine" and trust the Lord for how he will use me during this last season of life. My thoughts in this book are certainly a result of my efforts in retirement, knowing the Lord can continue to use them long after I'm gone.

A few months later as the area began to recover from COVID, I was able to help interview and select a "young" chaplain who could take my spot on the hospice team. I was honored when everyone told him he had big shoes to fill. I was grateful and knew my accomplishments were only a result of "Christ working through me to His honor and glory."

CHAPTER 34

---∞---

Attitude of Gratitude

Having an attitude of gratitude allows us to be content. Being grateful for what we have been given or blessed with allows God to bless us with a joy that only He can supply. With that attitude of gratitude, we can thank God for what he has given us (no matter how little or much), which brings us a God-given contentment. This idea is completely contrary to the "the grass is greener on the other side" philosophy or "the one who dies with the most toys wins."

The truth of God's word and His instructions for life are the foundation for a quality of life that only God can provide. Today, many individuals are ignorant of God's Word and are quickly going in the wrong direction with no moral compass.

Only the Creator God of this world is the writer for the instruction book of life. Trying to live without God's Word is like giving a model car with all the exact, scaled pieces to a child and telling him to put it together. The child has seen and ridden in many cars and is confident he knows how to put it together without instructions. The child may be able to figure out where the obvious pieces like the doors, wheels, and hood might go, but when they try to put together the detailed pieces of the engine and transmission, they will soon make a mess of the model. If they are wise enough, they will ask for help and know they need to follow the instruction book written by the model's creator.

Some people are like that child, thinking they have life all figured out and have a better way to do things than God. It remains to be seen if they are wise enough to come to the Creator of life for help to clean up their messes and then follow His instruction book, the Bible, to put the pieces of life together and make them all work as designed.

I'm Grateful for You

Thank you for taking the time to read my stories, insights, and thoughts. May the King of Kings and Lord of Lords use them to help make a small difference in your life. May you find the purpose He has created for you, and may He use every aspect of your life to His glory. May you find your life enriched as you work to be a blessing to others. As you read God's instruction book and are led by His Spirit, may He not only richly bless you but also guide you, enabling you to make every effort to make a difference in our world.

Numbers 6:24–26 (NLT)

May the LORD bless you and protect you.
May the LORD smile on you and be gracious to you.
May the LORD show you his favor and give you his peace.

Romans 15:13 (NLT)

I pray that God, the source of hope, will fill you completely with joy and peace because you trust in him. Then you will overflow with confident hope through the power of the Holy Spirit.

CHAPTER 35

————⋈————

Little Bursts of Meaningful Thought

I have always appreciated pithy Christian sayings that are like little bursts of meaningful thought. I like to use them often because they are reminders of truth that cause us to think on it. One that I was well known for repeating to our staff was: "Those who are flexible shall not be bent out of shape." It always seemed to get the point across that we need to be flexible or more fluid when confronted with change as opposed to what we thought would happen. Anytime our expectations are at a certain level, and the reality of life sets in, we can't help but be disappointed.

In the Bible that I carried for work, I collected many pithy sayings that were meaningful to me and I wanted to share them with you. Here they are. I hope they will be meaningful to you as well.

- When trouble grows, your character shows.
- Conscience is like a sundial; when the truth of God shines on it, it points in the right direction.

159

- "Let your conscience be your guide" is only valid if God's Word is guiding your conscience.
- Our faith may be tested so that we may trust His faithfulness.
- God provides redemption to any who repent, believe, and receive it.
- The storms of life prove the strength of our anchor.
- We walk a desert pathway, but the end of the journey is the Garden of God.
- Sin impacts blessing.
- When we see the world through the filter of God's Word, we learn the truth about both.
- The Bible doesn't keep us from knowing the truth; it prevents us from believing lies.
- Faith is our ability to see God in the dark.
- If you make room for Jesus in your heart, He will make room for you in heaven.
- The birth of Christ brought God to man. The cross of Christ brings man to God.
- Life's burdens are designed not to break us but to bend us toward God.
- Natural explanations are not final answers.
- When God gives us an impossible task, it becomes possible.
- Yesterday is gone; tomorrow is uncertain; today is here. Use it wisely.
- What matters is not faith and works; it is not faith or works; it is faith that works.
- The joys of heaven will more than compensate for the difficulties of life.
- Those who are flexible shall not be bent out of shape.

If this book has encouraged you, I'd love to hear from you. I can be reached at: falkenstinecraig@gmail.com.

———————⬦———————

CPSIA information can be obtained
at www.ICGtesting.com
Printed in the USA
BVHW030944280821
615448BV00007B/214

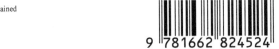